DR. MICHAEL HUNTER'S

BREAST DCIS

> **Hope** is the thing with feathers
> That perches in the soul
> And sings the tune without the words
> And never stops at all.
>
> Emily Dickinson

DR. MICHAEL HUNTER'S BREAST DCIS BOOK

© 2019 MICHAEL ANDREW HUNTER

All rights reserved, No portion of this book may be reproduced, stored in a retrieval system, or transmitted in any form or by any means - electronic, mechanical, photocopy, recording, scanning, or other - except for brief quotations in critical reviews or articles, without the prior written permission of the publisher.

PUBLISHED BY CANCERINFO, LLC

Any Internet addresses, phone numbers, or company or product information printed in this book are offered as a resource and are not intended in any way to be or to imply an endorsement by the publisher, nor does the publisher vouch for the existence, content, or services of these sites, phone numbers, companies, or products beyond the life of this book.

This book is not intended to provide therapy, counseling, or clinical advice or treatment, or to take the place of clinical advice and management from your personal health care provider. Readers are advised to consult their own qualified physicians regarding medical issues. Neither the publisher nor the author take any responsibility for any possible consequences from any treatment, action, or application of information in this book to the reader.

ISBN   9781080257638

Library of Congress Cataloging-in-Publication Data

Names: Hunter, Michael, author.
Title: Dr. Michael Hunter's Breast DCIS Book / Michael Hunter, M.D.

Subjects: DCIS Breast--Cancer--Epidemiology Breast--Cancer-Risk factors Breast--Cancer--DCIS -- Management

To everyone who wonders if I am writing for or about them in these pages. I am.

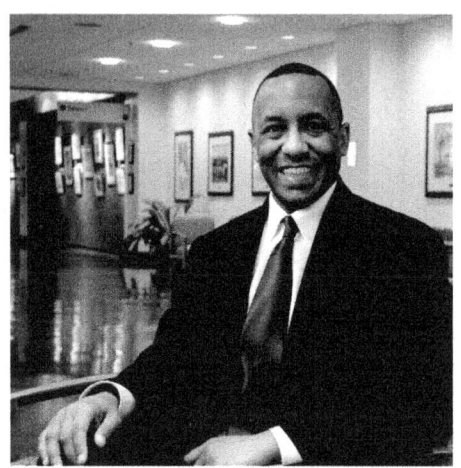

I am a **radiation oncologist** in Seattle (USA), and have degrees from Harvard, Yale, and University of Pennsylvania.

I have served on the Board of Komen Foundation of Puget Sound, as a consultant to the Washington Breast, Cervical, & Colon Health Project, and as cancer program medical director.

Michael Hunter MD

DR. MICHAEL HUNTER'S
BREAST DCIS BOOK

WWW.NEWCANCERINFO.COM

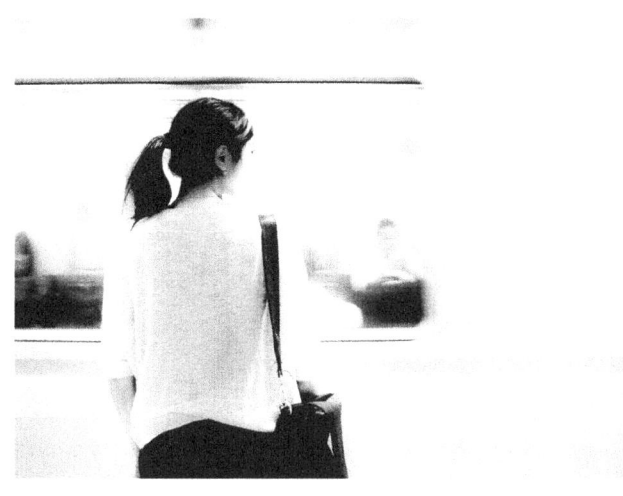

MY MISSION

Surreal. Few words have a greater impact. Many describe the time around hearing "You have breast cancer" as surreal, with many individuals moving from confusion to shock and grief, anger, fear, and despair. Most need time to work through these emotions. For those who have these feelings, once you work through them, you should be better able to navigate the journey to becoming more well.

Breast cancer is a story with many chapters. No matter where you find yourself in the journey, I designed this book to help you navigate it. Herein, you will find information about why you may have gotten breast ductal carcinoma *in situ* (and basic, sustainable lifestyle adjustments that might improve the odds of it never coming back), what it looks like under the microscope, staging (extent of cancer), prognosis, and management. For brevity, I will not focus on psychological well-being. I do hope to be a source of knowledge and support for you.

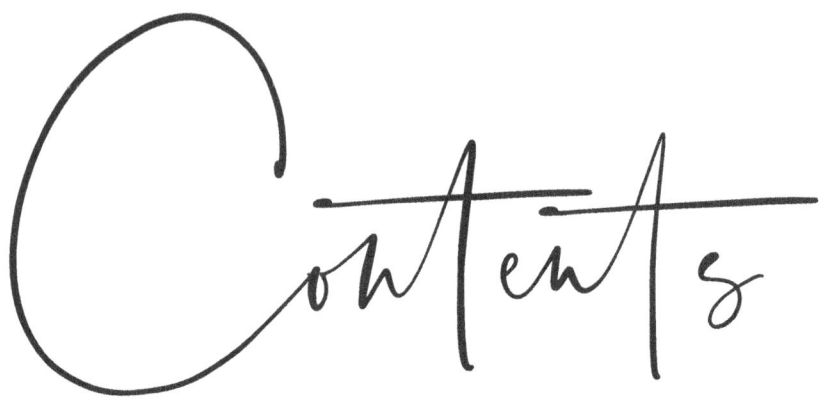

Basics	Image	Biopsy	Type	Stage
WHY?	MAMMO	TISSUE	DCIS	EXTENT
PAGE 13	PAGE 49	PAGE 81	PAGE 89	PAGE 127
1	**2**	**3**	**4**	**5**

	Manage	**Restore**	**Special**	**Survival**
	RELAPSE	PLASTICS	PAGET; YOUNG	AFTER
	PAGE 217	PAGE 223	PAGE 457	PAGE 457
	11	**12**	**13**	**14**

Chances	**Manage**	**Manage**	**Manage**	**Manage**
ODDS	PRE-SURGERY	SURGERY	RADIATION	ENDOCRINE
PAGE 141	PAGE 157	PAGE 169	PAGE 183	PAGE 203
6	**7**	**8**	**9**	**10**

BASICS

BREAST CANCER is the most common non-skin cancer among women worldwide. In 2018 in the USA, 266,120 cases of invasive breast cancer were diagnosed and 40,920 died of the disease. **Another 63,960 had non-invasive *(in situ)* disease.**

From the 1940s until the 1980s, breast cancer incidence (new cases) rates in the USA increased slightly. In the 1980s, incidence rose greatly (likely due to increased mammogram-based screening), and then leveled off during the 1990s. The incidence of breast cancer declined in the early 2000s. This decline appears to be linked to a drop in the use of menopausal hormone therapy (after the Women's Health Initiative study showed its use increased breast cancer risk). Since 2007, the incidence of breast cancer has remained roughly stable.

As the risk factors for non-invasive DCIS and invasive breast cancer are similar, I will address breast cancer in general in this first chapter.

MALE BREAST CANCER is uncommon. Still, in 2018, it is estimated that among men in the USA there were about 2.550 new cases, and 500 breast cancer deaths.

Inspire

Outcomes are improving

Mortality rates improving

Breast cancer death rates in the USA increased by 0.4 percent from 1975 to 1989, but thereafter decreased rapidly (for a total decline of 39 percent through 2015). The decrease occurred among younger and older women, but has slowed among women under 50 since 2007. This drop in mortality has been associated with improvements in treatment and early detection.

Not all groups have benefited from these advances equally: There has been a striking divergence in mortality trends among black and white women beginning in the early 1980s. As treatment improved, the gap between whites and blacks increased: In 2015, breast cancer death rates were 1.4 times higher among black American women, compared to their white counterparts.

Risk

While we cannot say with certainty why you (or someone about whom you care) got breast cancer, the disease is linked to many **risk factors.** We will review these in this chapter, but first I want to introduce some some key definitions:

- *Absolute risk*
  Odds you will develop a specific disease over a certain time

- *Lifetime risk*
  Odds you will develop a disease in your lifetime

- *Risk factors*
  Anything affecting your risk of getting a particular disease

- *Relative risk*
  Ratio of absolute risks

We will look at factors that are associated with a lower risk of getting breast cancer. We sometimes refer to such factors as protective risk facttors, or just protective factors.

RISK

You are told that if you take "anti-estrogen" pills (for example, tamoxifen) as a risk-reducing maneuver, your **relative risk** of breast cancer becomes about 0.5. This means that your risk of getting breast cancer is half that of someone in your situation who did not take the drug. On the other hand, a relative risk of 3 means that you are 3 times more likely to get a disease, compared to someone with a "normal" risk.

Numbers

Incidence

Ductal carcinoma *in situ* (DCIS) markedly increased from 5.8 per 100,000 women to 32.5 per 100,000 women in 2004, and then reached a plateau. This remarkable increase is largely due to utilization of breast cancer screening mammograms. In the United States, approximately 25 percent of breast cancers are DCIS, with an estimated 63,960 new cases of female breast cancer *in situ* found in 2018.

DCIS (a non-invasive form of breast cancer) is much less common than invasive breast cancer. Still, the risk factors for DCIS and invasive breast cancer are quite similar. Over the next several pages, we will review these risk factors, and also take a look at strategies you can employ to reduce your own personal risk of getting cancer in the future.

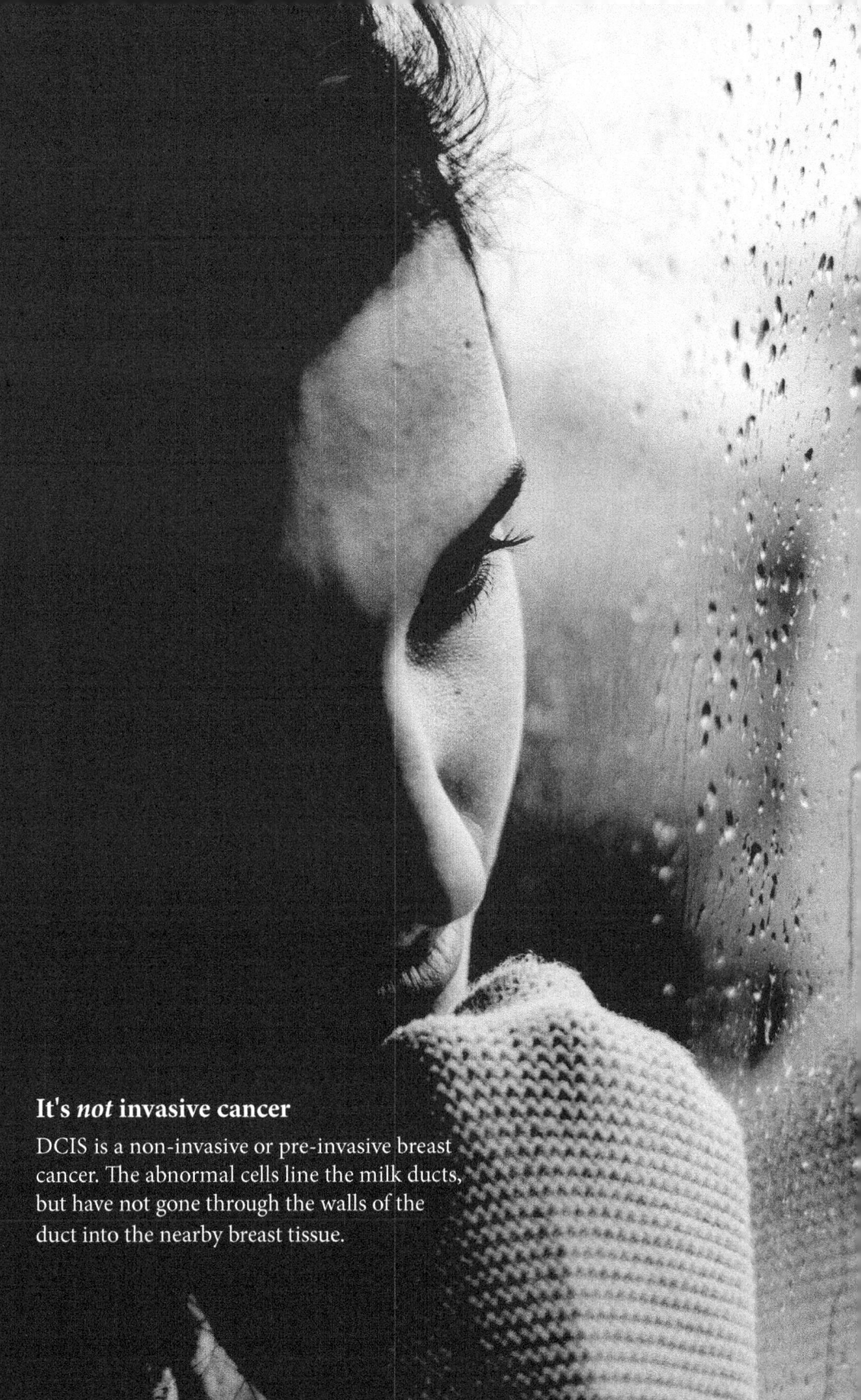

It's *not* invasive cancer

DCIS is a non-invasive or pre-invasive breast cancer. The abnormal cells line the milk ducts, but have not gone through the walls of the duct into the nearby breast tissue.

Why

"Fixed" risk factors

Age

Age is a risk factor for breast cancer among both women and men. **The older you are, the more likely you are to get breast cancer.** Less than five percent of women diagnosed with breast cancer in the USA are younger than age 40. About half of women with breast cancer will be diagnosed after 60 years of age. While the incidence of breast cancers driven by estrogen increases with age, the incidence of estrogen receptor-negative breast cancer increases until age 50, then levels off.

Female

Being a female is a strong risk factor for breast cancer. While men can get the breast cancer, the disease is approximately 100 times more common among women. However, the male incidence has risen slightly since 1975 (from 1 to 1.3 per 100,000). Men are more likely than women to be found with advanced-stage breast cancer, likely the result of lower awareness, and the lack of screening among men.

Personal history of breast cancer

A personal history of ductal carcinoma *in situ* (DCIS) or invasive breast cancer increases the risk of an invasive cancer in the opposite breast. This risk may be on the order of 0.5% per year, but this risk varies by factors such as your age at initial diagnosis, whether you have a so-called breast cancer gene (BRCA), and by the primary cancer hormone receptor status.

Height

The taller you are, the bigger your risk of getting breast cancer. In a study of over 100,000 women (followed for twelve years), women 5 feet 7 inches (1.75 meters) or taller were 1.57-times more likely to get breast cancer than women under 5 feet 2 inches (1.6 meters). Every 2 inches (5 centimeters) added 11 percent risk, or increased risk by a factor of 1.1.

AGE

RISK GENERALLY INCREASES WITH AGE

	RISK* over the next 10 years
20	1 in 1,567 (0.1%)
30	1 in 220 (0.5%)
40	1 in 68 (1.5%)
50	1 in 43 (2.3%)
60	1 in 29 (3.4%)
70	1 in 25 (3.9%)
Lifetime	**1 in 8 (12.4%)**

* your personal risk may be higher or lower

Density

Breast density describes the proportions of different breast tissue types. High breast density means that there is a greater amount of breast and connective tissue, as compared to breast fat. Low breast density means that there is a greater proportion of fat. High breast density is a risk factor for both invasive and non-invasive breast cancer. A pooled analysis of six studies found the positive association between breast density and DCIS risk to be largest for women under age 55.

Many (but not all) research studies demonstrate a link between breast density and the risk of getting breast cancer. Still, several states in the USA have enacted legislation mandating the reporting of breast density to women who have undergone mammography.

Geography

Breast cancer incidence rates around the world vary greatly. Developed countries (such as the United States, England and Australia) have higher rates than do developing countries (such as Cambodia, Nepal and Rwanda). **Incidence** worldwide is highest in Belgium, followed by Luxembourg, the Netherlands, France, New Caledonia (France), Lebanon, Australia, the United Kingdom, Italy, and New Zealand. Within the United States, incidence also varies:

- Higher
  New Hampshire, Connecticut, Massachusetts, Rhode Island, Delaware, New Jersey, Hawaii, Illinois, Minnesota, and New York

- Lower
  Wyoming, Nevada, New Mexico, Arizona, Texas, Utah, Florida, Oregon, Arkansas, and Mississippi

Mortality also varies by geography. While variations in mortality rates reflect variations in incidence, the other major contributor to the mortality rate is survival. Breast cancer mortality rates among white women tend to be highest in the North Central, Mid-Atlantic, and Western USA. Among African-American women, the highest death rates are found in some of the South Central and Mid-Atlantic states, as well as California. Some factors that may contribute to these differences include variations in risk factors, access to screening, and treatment. These are in turn influenced by socio-economic factors, legislative policies, and proximity to medical services.

Race

Among women in the USA, breast cancer incidence and mortality vary by race and ethnicity. Non-hispanic whites and African-Americans have the highest risk of getting breast cancer, followed by Latinas, Native Americans, Asians and Pacific Islanders. However, among women under 45, African-American incidence is the highest.

African-American women have the highest breast cancer-related death rate, while Asian-American and Pacific Islander women have the lowest. Between 2008 to 2012, rates of breast cancer diagnosis increased by 0.4 percent per year in African-American women, compared to 1.5 percent per year among women identifying as Asian or Pacific Islanders. The rates of diagnosis in the time period remained stable among women of white, Hispanic, American Indian and Alaska Native origins.

American Cancer Society researchers analyzed data from the National Cancer Institute's Surveillance, Epidemiology and End Results (SEER), and found that in 2012 black and white women were diagnosed with breast cancer at about the same rate. In seven states, the rates of breast cancer among black women surpassed the rates of white women between 2009 and 2012. That increase was seen primarily in the Southern region of the country: Alabama, Kentucky, Louisiana, Mississippi, Missouri, Oklahoma and Tennessee.

African-Americans - Incidence

The reasons for the rise in breast cancer incidence among African-Americans are not entirely clear, but some researchers suggest lifestyle factors might be primary factors. For example, being overweight is associated with a higher risk of getting breast cancer, at least for women who have completed menopause. Obesity rates among African-American women have increased substantially over time, from 39 percent in 1999 to 58 percent in the 2009 through 2012 period.

While obesity among the overall population of *post-menopausal* women is known to increase the chances of an individual getting breast cancer, there are a number of alternative explanations for this rise in breast cancer incidence among African-American women. However, the bottom line is that we do not know why with any certainty why African-Americans have a higher probability of dying of breast cancer.

African-Americans - Mortality

African-American women with breast cancer are 1.4-times more likely to die from their cancer compared with white women. While socioeconomic factors such as income, health insurance and access to health services are probable contributants to these disparities, they don't fully explain the different risks. Differences in rates of getting screening mammograms doesn't explain it either: African-American women and white women now have the same rates of mammogram use. In 2013, among women 40 and older, 66 percent of African-American women and 66 percent of white women had had a mammogram in the prior two years.

Investigators at the Harvard Massachusetts General Hospital assessed white and African-American women with stages I to III breast cancer diagnosed from 1988 to 2013. These women had their breast cancer tissue submitted to The Cancer Genome Atlas. The researchers then evaluated the association of race and genetic traits with tumor recurrence. Here is what they found:

African Americans as a group had greater genetic variation within a given tumor, and more basal gene expression tumors. This pattern suggests a **more aggressive tumor biology among African Americans** than among whites, a factor that may contribute to the significant racial disparities seen when examining breast cancer outcomes among different racial groups. In addition, socioeconomic and health care access disparities may contribute to worse outcomes among African American women.

Immigrants

Immigrants typically see a rise in their breast cancer incidence, after coming to the United States. For example, women who come to the United States from Asian countries (where breast cancer incidence is four to seven times lower than in the United States) experience a 1.8-times increase in risk after living in the USA a decade or more. A generation later, the risk for their daughters approaches that of USA-born women.

Turning to Latina women, those born in the United States have a significantly higher rate of breast cancer than do immigrant Latinas, but the longer the period of time immigrant women spend in the United States, the greater their risk for breast cancer. This is especially true for women who immigrate to the USA before the age of 20 years old.

Family

Most women with breast cancer *do not* have a family history of it. In fact, only about 13 percent have a first-degree relative (mother, sister or daughter) with breast cancer. However, a family history of certain cancers (for example breast, ovarian, or prostate cancer) can increase your risk of breast cancer.

- A first-degree relative (sister, mother, or daughter) has breast cancer: Your breast cancer risk may double.
- Two first-degree relatives have breast cancer: Your risk may triple.

Inherited genetics

Only 5 to 10 percent of all breast cancers are directly linked to the inheritance of known breast cancer susceptibility genes such as BRCA1, BRCA2, p53, ATM, and PTEN. Breast and ovarian cancer appear to be more common among women of Ashkenazi (with ancestors from Central or Eastern Europe) Jewish descent, given a higher prevalence of risk-raising BRCA1 and BRCA2 (BReast CAncer genes 1 and 2) mutations.

Everyone has BRCA1 and BRCA2 genes. Alas, some have an inherited mutation in one or both of these genes that increases the risk of several cancer. One in 40 women of Ashkenazi Jewish descent carry one of these mutations, compared to one in 400 in the general population. Of those with breast cancer, roughly 10 percent will have a BRCA mutation. Among women with breast cancer in the non-Ashkenazi Jewish population, about five percent carry a BRCA mutation.

Are BRCA mutations limited to individuals of Askenazi Jewish descent? Clearly, the answer is no; various ethnic and racial groups are susceptible as well. For example, young African-American women with a breast cancer diagnosis at age 50 years or younger have a much higher BRCA mutation frequency than that previously reported among young white women with breast cancer, according to a recent United States-based study.

Women with inherited mutations in the BRCA genes are significantly more likely to develop breast or ovarian cancer, especially at a younger age. About 5% of women with breast cancer in the United States have mutations in a BRCA1 or BRCA2 gene, based on estimates among non-Hispanic white women. Having a BRCA gene mutation can raise your risk of several cancer types, including melanoma, as well as ovarian and other gynecologic cancers, breast (including among males), pancreas, prostate cancer, and other solid tumors..

Other genetic factors

• P53 / Li-Fraumeni syndrome
p53 gene mutations can raise your risk of breast cancer, leukemia, and cancers of the lung and brain. Those with Li-Fraumeni syndrome have a 50% risk of breast cancer by the age of 60, and p53 mutations may be associated with up to 7% of all breast cancers among women under age 40. These cancers tend to be estrogen, progesterone, and HER2 receptor positive.

• PTEN/Cowden syndrome (uncommon)
The PTEN gene provides instructions for making an enzyme found in almost all tissues. The enzyme acts as a tumor suppressor; it helps regulate cell division by keeping cells from growing and dividing too rapidly or in an uncontrolled way. PTEN gene mutations can lead to the growth of numerous hamartomas (a benign, non-cancer growth), and can increase the risk of thyroid, uterus, and breast cancer. Those who have it have a lifetime breast cancer risk of up to 85%.

• More
Other gene abnormalities have been linked with an increased risk of breast cancer. Mutations in ATM, BRIP1, CHEK2, NBS1, PALB2, and RAD50 are linked to a 2- to 4-fold increase in breast cancer risk. These genes are typically low penetrance (less likely to show), and contribute less to the overall numbers of breast cancer, at least compared to BRCA, p53, or PTEN mutations.

Tobacco
Some studies point to tobacco use as slightly raising the risk of breast cancer.

For example, the EPIC study found a 1.06-fold increase in risk at 11 years follow-up, while the Nurses' Health Study demonstrated a 1.09-fold increase at the 30 year follow-up mark. Meta-analyses (analyses of collections of studies) show mixed results: The Collaborative Group on Hormonal Factors in Breast Cancer demonstrated no increase in breast cancer risk. On the other hand, two other meta-analyses found a 1.12 to 1.13-fold increase in risk.

DES (diethylstilbestrol)
Some pregnant women in the USA received the drug DES between 1940 and 1971 to reduce the risk of miscarriage. Women who took DES during pregnancy have a slightly elevated risk of breast cancer. Women who were exposed to DES in utero - that is, whose mothers took DES while pregnant - may have a slightly increased risk of breast cancer after age 40.

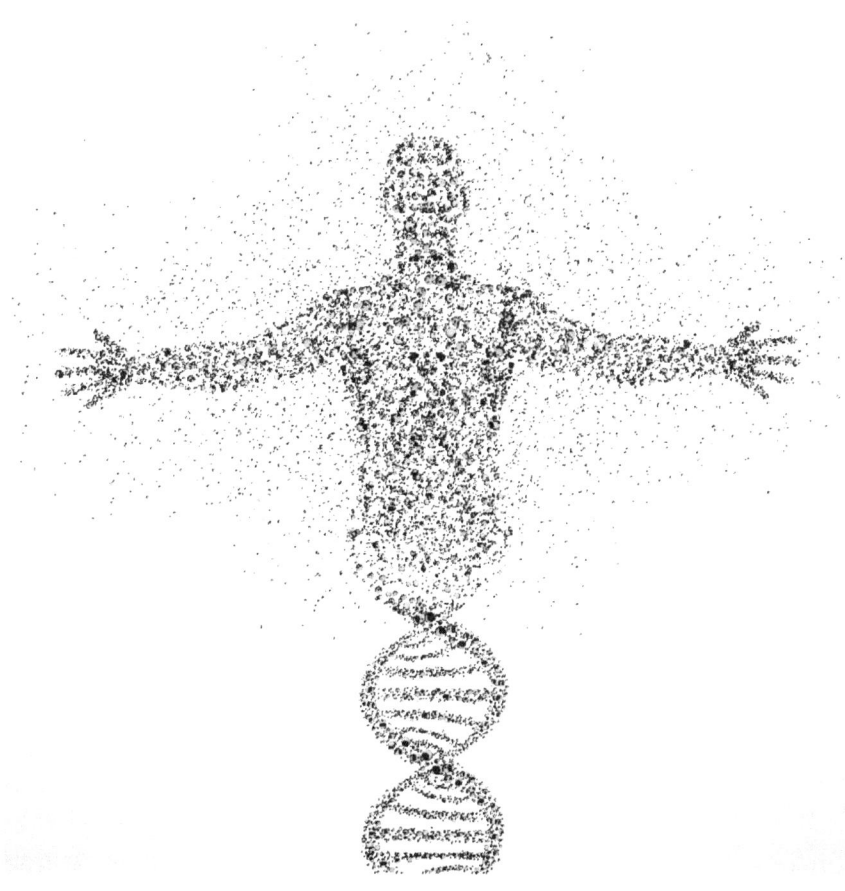

Usually *not* inherited genetics

Only 5 to 10 percent of breast cancers are directly linked to the inheritance of known breast cancer susceptibility genes.

Hyperplasia and other benign breast conditions

Benign breast conditions are not cancers, but some increase your risk of getting breast cancer, and others do not.

- Proliferative (fast-growing cells) increase risk

    Usual hyperplasia: May double breast cancer risk, compared to women without a proliferative disorder.

    Atypical (ductal or lobular) hyperplasia (ADH; ALH): May increase breast cancer risk by a factor of four or five, compared to women without a proliferative condition. Women with atypical hyperplasia may consider taking a risk-lowering drug such as tamoxifen or raloxifene.

- Non-proliferative (cells not fast-growing) don't increase risk, unless nearby cells are atypical or DCIS. Non-proliferative conditions include simple cysts, fibroademonas, and intraductal papillomas. Some studies have found radial scars increase risk, while other have not.

LCIS

When abnormal cells grow inside the breast lobules, but have not spread to nearby tissue or beyond, the condition is called lobular carcinoma *in situ* (LCIS). *In situ* means "remaining in place." In spite of containing the term carcinoma (cancer), **lobular carcinoma *in situ* is not itself a cancer.** However, LCIS can markedly increase your risk of developing a breast cancer in the future, in either breast. LCIS does not cause symptoms and typically does not show up on a mammogram. It tends to be found as a result of a biopsy performed on the breast for some other reason.

The finding of **LCIS is associated with a 30 to 40 percent lifetime risk** of developing an invasive breast cancer. This compares to a risk of approximately 12.5 percent for a woman at average risk in the USA. Another study puts the breast cancer risk at 21 percent over the ensuing 15 years. Management options for those with LCIS may include anti-estrogen drugs such as tamoxifen, removal of both breasts, or incorporation of MRI with mammograms for high-risk screening.

Diabetes

The risk of developing breast cancer varies by diabetes type:

Type 1 (insulin-dependent; juvenile) diabetes*: No increase in risk
- Typically occurs before the age of 40
- The body doesn't produce insulin
- Type 1 diabetes *does not* increase breast cancer risk.

Type 2 diabetes: Increased breast cancer risk
- The body does not produce enough insulin to function properly, or the cells in the body do not react normally to the insulin it does produce (insulin resistance).
- Risk factors for Type 2 diabetes include being overweight, physically inactive and eating an unhealthy diet.
- Type 2 diabetes *increases* breast cancer risk: Postmenopausal women 50 years or older who have type 2 diabetes have about a 1.2 to 1.27-fold increase in risk of developing breast cancer. We don't fully understand why breast cancer risk is increased, but many risk factors are similar for type 2 diabetes and for breast cancer.

Gestational (pregnancy-related) diabetes: No increase in risk
- The body is unable to produce enough insulin to transfer all of the glucose into cells, causing high blood glucose levels.
- Most can control their diabetes with exercise and diet.
- Gestational diabetes is *not* itself linked to an increase in breast cancer risk. But, while blood glucose levels usually go back to normal after pregnancy, there is a 35 to 65 percent chance of developing type 2 diabetes in the next 10-20 years.

Thyroid cancer

There *may* be an association between thyroid cancer and breast cancer incidence: Several lines of evidence suggest that breast cancer and thyroid cancer occur together in the same female patients more frequently than would be expected by chance. While I would not recommend routine screening for thyroid cancer among those with breast cancer, it seems reasonable to *emphasize* routine breast cancer screening among those with thyroid cancer.

Risk factors

Hormone-related

Early menarche

Early age at menstrual period onset (menarche) is linked associated with a higher risk. There is a one-tenth reduction in risk for every two year delay in the menses onset. The average age of menarche in the USA is 13 (slightly higher for Asians, and slightly lower for Hispanics and African-Americans).

Late menopause

A pooled analysis of more than 400,000 women found that for every year older a woman was at menopause, breast cancer risk increased by three percent. A woman who enters menopause after 55 years of age has twice the risk of a woman who did so before 45.

No children

Women who have not had a full-term pregnancy have a 1.2 to 1.7-fold increase in risk. A full-term pregnancy reduces your total number of lifetime menstrual cycles. In addition, breast cells are immature and very active until your first full-term pregnancy. The immature breast cells respond to the hormone estrogen: Your first full-term pregnancy makes the breast cells more fully mature, with the cells then growing in a more regular way. Immediately following a full-term pregnancy, a woman's risk of getting breast cancer actually *increases*. By a decade later, the pregnancy begins to reduce risk. The initial increase is especially true among women over 35, with a 1.26-fold increase in risk 5 years after delivery.

Increasing age of first full-term pregnancy

Women who become pregnant later in life are at increased risk of developing breast cancer. The cumulative risk (as compared to women with a full-term pregnancy, up to age 70) is 20% lower, 10% lower, and 5% higher among women who delivered their first child at age 20, 25, or 35 years, respectively.

Modifiable: Reproductive

Birth control pills

If you are currently using birth control pills (or stopped recently), you may have a 1.2 to 1.3-fold increased risk of breast cancer (compared to women who never used oral contraceptives). Once a woman stops taking birth control pills, her risk begins to decrease. By a decade or so later, the risk becomes similar to a woman who has never been on the pill. However, most studies are older, and looked at the use of higher-dose forms of birth control pills. Research continues on more modern forms of the pill, and some forms (mini-pills) may not have an increased risk. In addition, birth control pills may *reduce* your risk of uterus and ovarian cancer, in addition to reducing the chances of undesired pregnancy. Data regarding Depo Provera, hormone-releasing IUDs, birth control patches and vaginal ring are limited.

Breast-feeding

Breast-feeding lowers breast cancer risk, especially among premenopausal women. A pooled analysis of 47 studies examining *cumulative* time spent breast-feeding yielded the following results, noting that while studies show breast cancer risk is lower among women who have breast-fed, few studies have looked at associations between breast-feeding and a lower risk of particular types of breast cancer. For those who breast feed less than a year, risk reduction is possible. Breast feed a year, and risk slightly decreases, with two years' duration giving twice the benefit as one year. Breast feeding more than two years provides the most risk reduction.

Hormone receptor-negative breast cancers have no receptors for the hormones estrogen or progesterone (they are estrogen- and progesterone receptor negative). This subtype of breast cancer doesn't respond to hormonal medicines which target hormone receptors, and is considered more aggressive than hormone receptor-positive breast cancer. A meta-analysis (a study that combines and analyzes the results of a number of earlier studies) found that women who had breast-fed for any amount of time had an up to 20 percent lower risk of developing hormone receptor-negative breast cancer. The association between breast-feeding and receptor-positive breast cancers needs more investigation.

Other risk factors

Light at night, melatonin and breast cancer

Melatonin is a hormone that helps regulate your sleep cycle. At night, we produce more melatonin, leading to sleep. Exposure to light at night can suppress the melatonin production. Lowering melatonin increases estrogen, potentially increasing your breast cancer risk.

Radiation exposure in youth

Significant radiation exposure early in life (for example, radiation therapy to the chest area for a childhood cancer) increases the breast cancer risk significantly. If you have had therapeutic irradiation to the chest region, ask a valued healthcare professional about recommended screening for you. Later in this chapter, we will turn to some potential risk-reducing maneuvers.

Hormone replacement therapy (HRT)

- **Combination estrogen/progesterone**

Breast cancer risk increases within the first five years of use of combination estrogen/progesterone use. The risk goes up each year a woman takes estrogen plus progestin; use for five or more years (and current) more than doubles risk. After use stops, risk begins to drop. After 5 to 10 years, risk returns to that of a woman who has never used hormone replacement therapy (HRT).

- **Estrogen alone**

Estrogen may increase risk *after* 10 to 20 years of use: While the Women's Health Initiative (WHI) trial showed a *decreased* risk of breast cancer with estrogen alone compared to placebo after an average of seven years of use, more recent studies suggest the use of estrogen alone may increase breast cancer risk after ten to 20 years of use.

HORMONE REPLACEMENT
RISK WITH ESTROGEN + PROGESTERONE

	Extra cases per 10,000 women
Breast cancer	9
Deep vein thrombosis (clots)	4
Pulmonary embolism (lung clots)	4
Stroke	5

	Fewer cases per 10,000 women
Uterus (endometrial) cancer	3
Hip fracture	5

The Women's Health Initiative (WHI) study, which demonstrated the association between menopausal hormone replacement therapy and invasive breast cancer, also reported on associations with DCIS. While not statistically significant, the DCIS results were in the same direction as the results for invasive breast cancer, **suggesting that estrogen plus progesterone may be associated with an increased risk of DCIS.**

Changeable: Estrogen-related factors

Weight gain after menopause increases risk

Before menopause, extra weight is protective, as blood levels of estrogen are lower among those who are overweight. Being overweight becomes harmful *after* menopause: The risk for getting breast cancer may be up to nearly 1.6-times higher than for normal-weight post-menopausal women. In one recent study, researchers found that post-menopausal women who were overweight/obese had an increased invasive breast cancer risk compared with women of normal weight, with greater risk associated with severe obesity. Very obese women had an increased risk for estrogen- and progesterone-driven breast cancer, but *not* for other types. These women were also at increased risk for larger tumors and death. Women with a baseline Body Mass Index (BMI) of under 25 who gained more than 5% of their body weight over the years of the study also had an increased risk for breast cancer. However, women already overweight or obese did not.

Alcohol

Alcohol consumption increases the cancer risk in general: In 1988, the International Agency for Research on Cancer (IARC) declared that **alcohol is a carcinogen.** A recent study showed a dose-response relationship exists between alcohol consumption and the risk of getting breast cancer among both pre- and post-menopausal women. In the European Prospective Investigation Into Cancer and Nutrition (EPIC) study, 334,850 women ages 35 to 70 were recruited in ten European countries and followed for an average of 11 years. Here are the results:

- Alcohol was associated with risk: Each 10 gram/day increase in alcohol intake raised risk by 4.2%.
- Risk was elevated for *both* hormone receptor-positive and hormone receptor-negative breast cancers.
- Risk was higher among women who started drinking before their first full-term pregnancy.

Current evidence is sufficient to conclude that alcohol is causally related to the development of breast cancer.

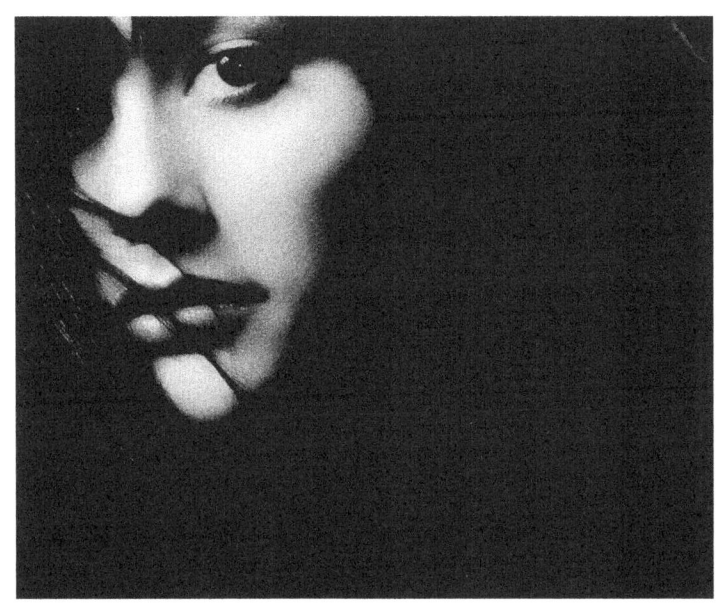

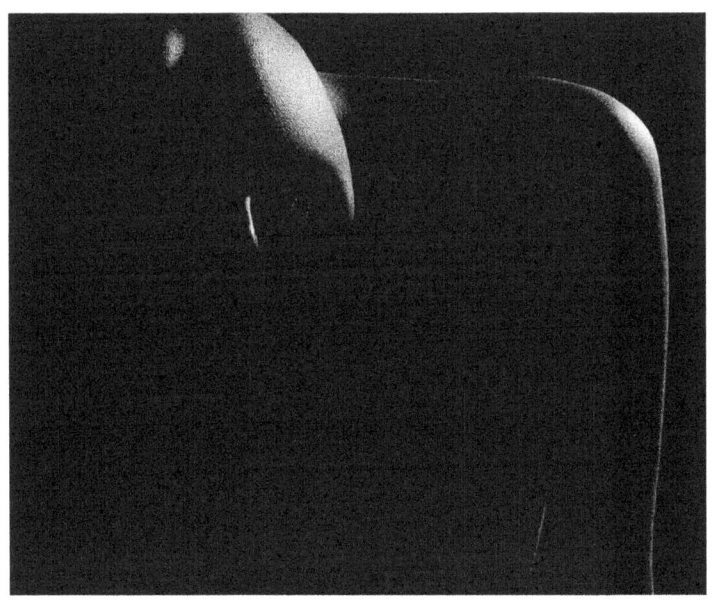

Changeable: Diet

Mediterranean Diet

A Mediterranean diet (rich with plant foods, fish and olive oil) is associated with better heart health. A Spanish study suggests it *may* also reduce the risk of developing breast cancer. Investigators randomly assigned more than 4,200 women, ages 60 to 80, to eat either a Mediterranean diet supplemented with extra virgin olive oil or with nuts, versus a low-fat control diet. The women, who joined the study in 2003 to 2009 were all at high risk for heart disease, and their average body mass index was 30 (considered obese; obesity is itself a risk factor for the development of post-menopausal breast cancer). Less than 3 percent had used hormone therapy, and the average age was 68.

Compared with the control diet group, the **Mediterranean plus olive oil group had a 68 percent lower risk of developing breast cancer** over a five year follow-up period. While the Mediterranean diet with nuts reduced risk, the results were not statistically significant. There are some limitations to the study, including the fact that breast cancer was *not* the primary subject of the research. In addition, it is unclear whether the olive oil was beneficial on its own, or only when taken with the Mediterranean diet.

How much olive oil?

Women in the study consumed four tablespoons daily, using it as a spread, for salads, and for cooking. Those in the nut consumption group ate about an ounce of nuts daily, half walnuts and the other half split between hazelnuts and almonds. While the results seem promising, we need longer follow-up, and validation studies. Still, this PREDIMED study adds to growing support for the health benefits of a Mediterranean-type diet.

A systematic review suggests the Mediterranean dietary pattern (and diets composed largely of vegetables, fruit, fish, and soy) is associated with a decreased risk of breast cancer. Researchers found no association between traditional dietary patterns and the risk of getting breast cancer, and only one study showed a significant increase in risk associated with the Western dietary pattern. For those who already have breast cancer, I am unaware of an effect of any particular diet on prognosis, but generally suggest adherence to a balanced diet, including copious fruits and vegetables (and not much red meat).

Lower fat diet

The federally funded Women's Health Initiative (WHI) clinical trial of dietary modification in nearly 49,000 **postmenopausal** women with no previous history of breast cancer reported that women who followed a balanced diet that was low in fat and included daily servings of fruits, vegetables, and grains had a 21% lower risk of death from breast cancer than women in the control group who continued their normal diet, which was higher in fat overall. This is the first large, randomized clinical trial to show that diet can reduce the risk of dying from breast cancer. Researchers presented these remarkable results at the 2019 ASCO Annual Meeting in Chicago (USA).

The study enrolled 48,835 post-menopausal women age 50 to 79 with no previous breast cancer history. From 1993 to 1998, researchers randomly assigned women to their normal diet (where fat accounted for 32% or more of their daily calories), or a diet with the **goal of reducing fat consumption to 20% or less of caloric intake as well as requiring at least one serving of a vegetable, fruit, and grain in their daily diets.** Women in the balanced, low-fat diet group adhered to the diet for approximately 8.5 years. The investigators continued to follow all of these women after completion of the intervention period to see if they died from any cause or from breast cancer.

There was a 15% lower risk of death from any cause after a breast cancer diagnosis in the balanced, low-fat diet group. **There was a 21% lower risk of death solely from breast cancer in the balanced, low-fat diet group.** Here is the view of the lead investigator:

> "Ours is the first randomized, controlled trial to prove that a healthy diet can reduce the risk of death from breast cancer," offered Rowan Chlebowski, MD, PhD, FASCO, from the Los Angeles Biomedical Research Institute at Harbor-UCLA Medical Center in Torrance, California. "The balanced diet we designed is one of moderation, and after nearly 20 years of follow-up, the health benefits are still accruing."

Changeable: Blue light at night

Exposure to light

Light at night is bad for your health, and exposure to blue light emitted by electronics and energy-efficient light bulbs may be especially so. Here is an excerpt from the *Harvard Health Letter*:

> "Until the advent of artificial lighting, the sun was the major source of lighting, and people spent their evenings in (relative) darkness. Now, in much of the world, evenings are illuminated, and we take our easy access to all those lumens for granted. But we may be paying a price for basking in all that light. At night, light throws the body's biological clock—the circadian rhythm—out of whack. Sleep suffers. Worse, research shows that it may contribute to the causation of cancer, diabetes, heart disease, and obesity."

Night shift

Many (but certainly not all) studies have linked working night shift to a higher risk of breast and prostate cancer, diabetes, heart disease, and obesity. It's not entirely clear why night time light exposure seems to be so bad for us. We do know that exposure to light drops your melatonin, a hormone that influences our awake/sleep rhythms. There is some very early evidence that lower melatonin levels might explain the association with cancer.

Type of light: The blues

Melatonin is a hormone in your body that plays a role in sleep. The production and release of melatonin in the brain is connected to time of day, increasing when it's dark and decreasing when it's light. Melatonin production declines with age. While light of any color can suppress melatonin, blue light/wavelengths (beneficial during daylight hours because they boost attention, reaction times, and mood) seem to be the most disruptive at night. Exposure to electronics with screens (and energy-efficient lighting) is increasing our exposure to blue wavelengths, especially after sundown. Harvard researchers examined the effects of 6.5 hours of blue light exposure with exposure to green light of comparable brightness. The blue light suppressed melatonin for about twice as long as the green light and shifted the natural 24 hour cycle by twice as much (3 hours vs. 1.5 hours).

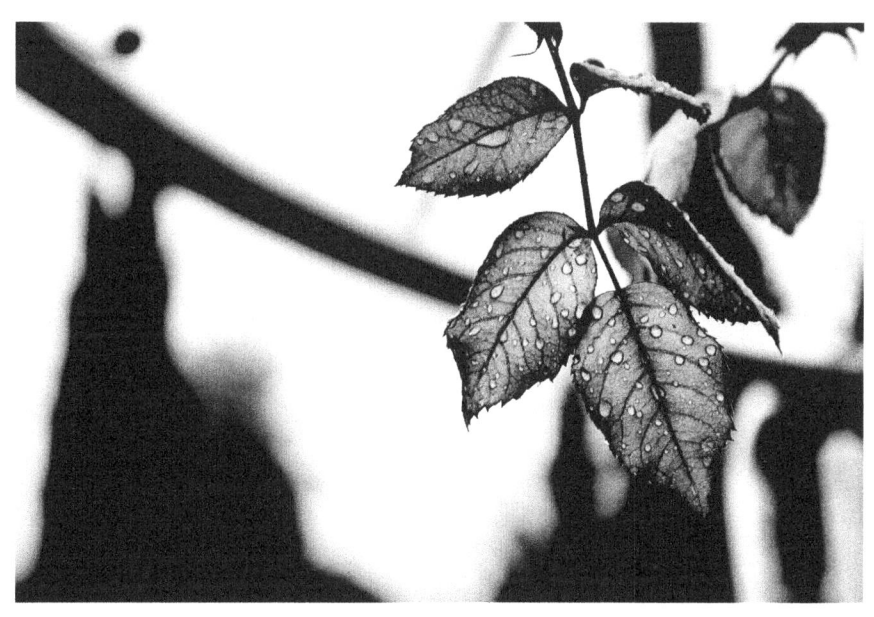

Changeable: Lifestyle

Physical Activity

Physical activity may lower the risk of breast cancer, especially for women who have gone through menopause. Exercise can lower estrogen levels, fight obesity and boost immune system cells that attack tumors.

- Before you start an exercise program, please consult a valued health care provider. This is especially important if you have been inactive for a long time, are overweight, have a high risk of heart disease, or have a high risk of other chronic health problems.
- **Include physical activity in your daily routine.** Aim for the minimum of the equivalent of a brisk walk for 30 minutes daily.

Weight

- Gaining weight after menopause increases breast cancer risk.
- Weight gain of 20 pounds or more after the age of 18 *may* increase your risk of breast cancer.
- If you have gained weight, losing weight may lower your risk of breast cancer. Aim for a body mass index (BMI) of 20 to 25.

Breast feeding

Breast feeding can *lower* risk.

Alcohol

Having one serving of alcohol (for example, a glass of red wine) each day *may* improve your health by reducing your risk of heart disease and stroke. However, alcohol can increase your breast cancer risk: The more you drink, the higher your risk of developing breast cancer. If you drink alcohol, aim for less than one standard drink a day, on average. Getting enough folic acid may lower the risk linked to drinking alcohol, but the evidence here is not high-level. You can find folic acid in multivitamins, oranges, orange juice, green vegetables and fortified breakfast cereals.

RISKS

	Lower	Higher	RR*
BRCA mutation	Negative	Positive	3 to 7x increase
Mother/sister with breast cancer	No	Yes	2.6
Age	30 to 34	70 to 74	18
Age at menarche	Over 14	Less than 12	1.5
Age at first birth	Under 20	Over 30	1.9 to 3.5
Age at menopause	Under 45	Over 55	2
Use of contraceptive pills	Never	Past/current	1.1 to 1.2
Estrogen + progestin	Never	Current	1.2
Alcohol	None	2 to 5/day	1.4
Breast density	0	75 or higher	1.8 to 6
Bone density	Lowest quartile	Highest quartile	2.7 to 3.5
History of benign breast biopsy		Yes	1.7
History of atypical hyperplasia	No	Yes	3.7

Protective

Breast feeding (months)	16 or more	0	0.7
Full-term pregnancies	5 or more	0	0.7
Exercise	Yes	No	0.7
Postmenopausal BMI	Under 22.9	Over 30.7	0.6
Ovaries removed before age 35	Yes	No	0.3
Aspirin	More than once per week, 6+ months	Non-user	0.8

* relative risk

Breast cancer risk

Tools

Risk assessments are designed to educate patients about cancer risk, determine if genetic testing is indicated, and help decide when breast cancer screening with mammograms should start. High-risk patients can be offered screening breast magnetic resonance imaging (MRI) in addition to annual mammograms and chemoprevention to help reduce breast cancer risk,

Various risk-prediction models have been created for breast cancer. We may conveniently stratify women into one of three risk groups for the development of breast cancer:

- **Average risk (75% of women):** No family history of the disease and no significant personal risk factors (for example, a previous biopsy of the breast) that would constitute a higher risk. Those in the average risk group have a 12% chance of developing breast cancer.

- **Women with hereditary breast cancer** risk and a genetic mutation known to confer a high lifetime risk (12% of women).

- **Moderate risk:** Women with a family history of breast cancer not associated with known genes, or women who have had a breast biopsy that shows a precancerous change.

There are several credible online tools available to help women and their care providers better understand breast cancer risk. Such knowledge may help inform your decision-making regarding breast cancer risk reduction strategies, genetic counseling/testing options, and screening options for the earlier detection of breast cancer. Alas, there is no tool that can predict with certainty your indivual risk, and each test has both strengths and limitations. Let's look at some of these tools.

Risk assessment tool for the general public

Your Disease Risk *(www.yourdiseaserisk.wustl.edu)* is a wonderful website from Washington University (USA) that offers both educational material and a risk assessment tool for breast cancer (and other diseases as well). It puts you into above average, average, or below average risk categories, compared to the general population. I really like this relatively easy to use tool. The tool was developed using data for the USA, and estimates your risk relative to the US general population. In addition, the tool only considers limited information about your family history of breast cancer, which could lead to underestimating risk for some patients.

Risk assessment tools for health professionals

Many of these tools are accessible to you online. Still, if you choose to explore any of them, please discuss your results with a valued health care provider.

What	Factors	Notes
Gail model	Previous breast biopsies (and whether atypia is present); reproductive history (age at start of menstruation and age at first live birth of a child); family history of breast cancer among first-degree relatives (e.g. mother; sister; daughter)	• Only considers limited info about family breast cancer history • Does not include factors such as use of hormone replacement therapy, breast density, and lifestyle factors such as smoking, alcohol use, diet, or physical inactivity
Breast Cancer Risk Assessment Tool	Age; age at first menarche; age at first live birth of a child; family and personal history of breast cancer;	• A 5-year risk of 1.67% or higher is considered high risk for developing breast cancer
IBIS (Tyrer-Cuzick) Breast Cancer Risk Evaluation Tool	Age; age at first live birth of a child; age at first period; age at menopause; height and weight; prior risk-increasing benign biopsy of breast; use of hormones; comprehensive family history	• Does not include risk factors associated with lifestyle or breast density Genetic counseling advised when the model predicts a 10% or higher chance that you have a mutation of BRCA

At high risk?

Prophylactic bilateral mastectomy

Today, many high-risk women are choosing to have surgical removal of both breasts as a means of reducing their risk of developing breast cancer in the future. While such a radical move indeed reduces the risk, it remains unclear as to whether it has a significant impact on survival odds. Still, some choose removal of both breasts as they feel the complications associated with the surgery are worth the benefits (psychological; desire for symmetry; reduced need for future mammogram surveillance).

The primary goal of bilateral prophylactic (risk-reducing) mastectomy is to reduce breast cancer risk. Here are estimated risks, based on various factors:

Genetic risk factors	Lifetime risk
BRCA1	81%
BRCA2	85%
p53	24%
PTEN	25%

Non-genetic risk factors	Relative risk
Classic LIN*	7 to 11x
ADH/ALH*	4 to 5x
Proliferative change, without atypia	1.9x

* LIN lobular intraepithelial neoplasia
  ADH atypical ductal hyperplasia
  ALH atypical lobular hyperplasia

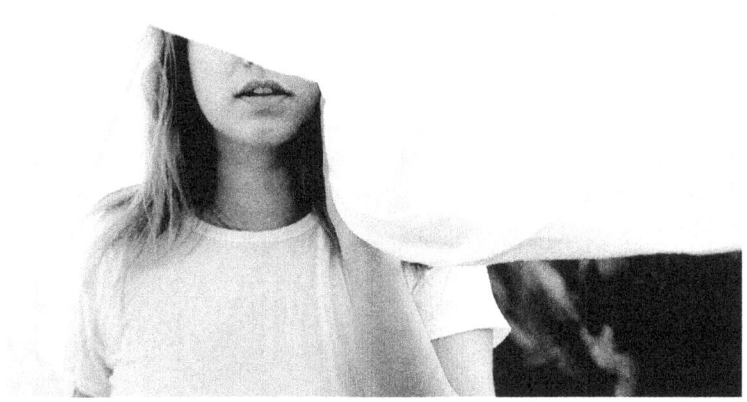

High risk? Consider:

	Relative risk drop
Tamoxifen (pills)	37-49%
Raloxifene (pills)	56-59%
Exemestane (pills)	65%
Removal of both ovaries	53%
Removal of both breasts	90-100%

A recent randomized trial of low-dose tamoxifen to prevent local and contralateral recurrence in breast intraepithelial neoplasia (atypical hyperplasia and lobular or ductal carcinoma *in situ*) showed tamoxifen at 5 milligrams daily for 3 years cut the recurrence of breast intraepithelial neoplsia in half, with a limited toxicity.

Key points

Risk

Breast cancer remains the most common (non-skin) cancer among women in the United States. Fortunately, mortality from breast cancer continues to decline. We may conveniently divide risk factors into one of three major groups:

- Inherited genetics
- Hormone-related (including reproductive factors)
- Environmental

Action list

Many risk factors are not easily modifiable. Still, let's focus on the ones that are potentially changeable:

- **Physical activity:** Aim for the equivalent of a brisk walk for 150 minutes per week (for example, 30 minutes for 5 days per week)

- **Weight:** Shoot for a Body Mass Index (BMI) of 20 to 25

- **Alcohol:** Be prudent, limiting consumption to no more than 3 to 7 standard drinks per week (and not more than 3 at any given time)

- **Diet:** Preferred diets include ones that are relatively low and fat, and rich in fruits and vegetables. Incorporate extra virgin olive oil into your diet, perhaps as much as 4 tablespoons per day!

- **Anti-estrogen (endocrine) therapy:** If you are on these pills, don't forget to take them as prescribed.

- **Hormones:** Combined long-term use of estrogen and progestin menopausal hormone replacement therapy increases breast cancer risk.

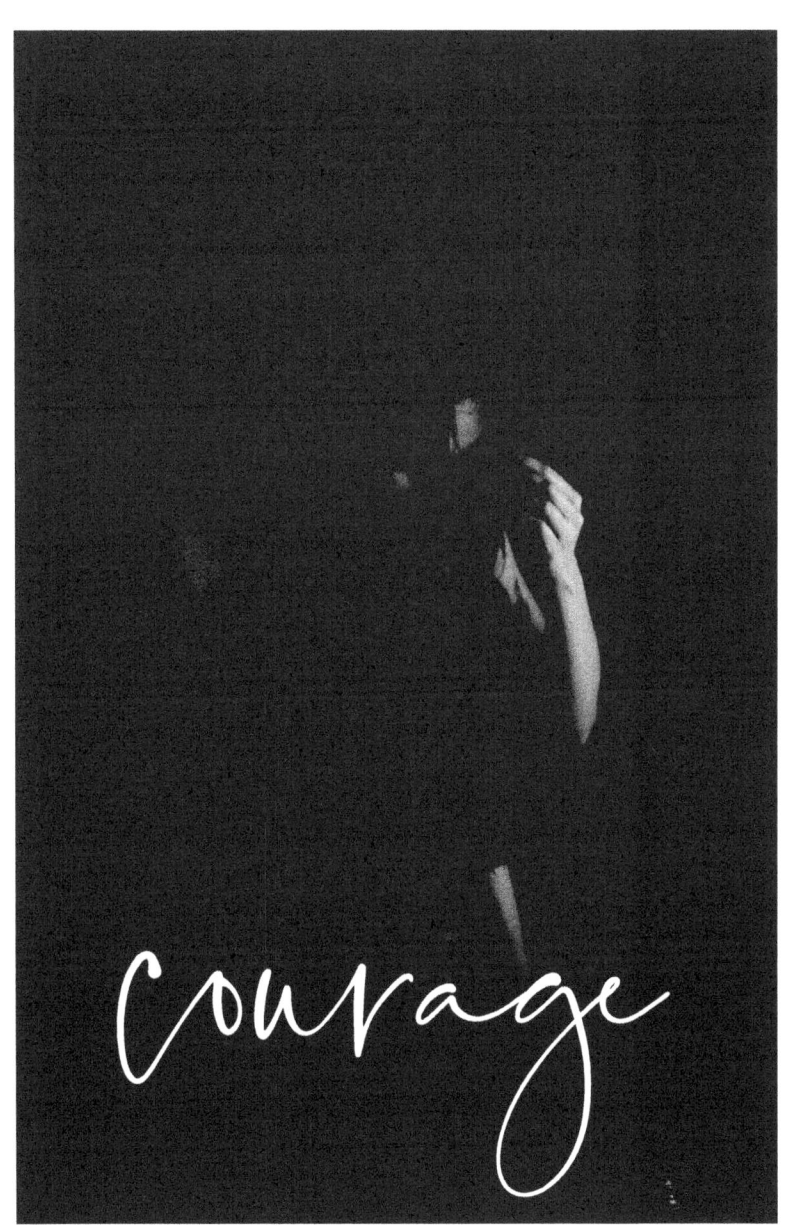

IMAGE

Tools

mam•mo•gram Images of the breast, obtained using X-rays.

Mammograms are the foundation of screening for women at average risk of getting the disease. Several randomized trials comparing screening mammograms versus no screening mammograms have shown that this imaging test decreases the odds of dying from breast cancer. Digital mammograms and tomosynthesis (3D mammograms) are more recent innovations.

ul•tra•sound Images of the breast, obtained using sound waves.

Ultrasound is commonly used as a diagnostic follow-up when there is something concerning on mammograms. While not generally used as a screening tool for women at average risk, Some centers will incorporate ultrasound into screening for highly select women with increased breast density.

MRI Images of the breast, obtained using powerful magnets.

Magnetic resonance imaging (MRI) is used for breast cancer diagnosis and staging. In addition, MRI may be used as a screening tool for women at higher risk. Breast MRI uses magnetic fields and an intravenous (IV) contrast agent to create images of the breast.

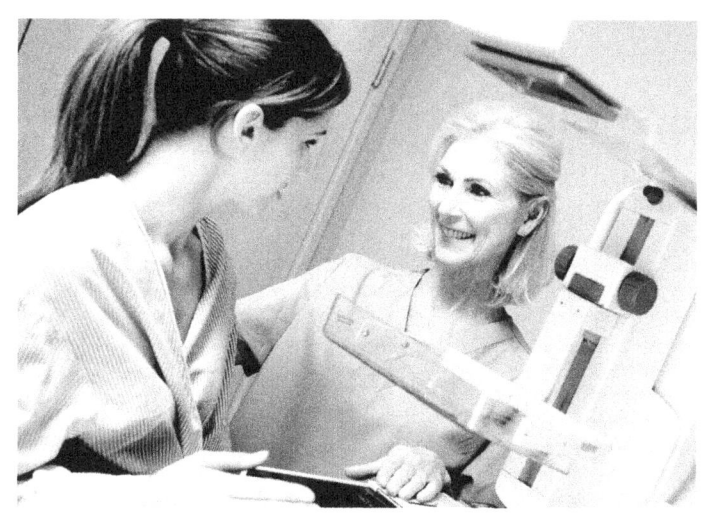

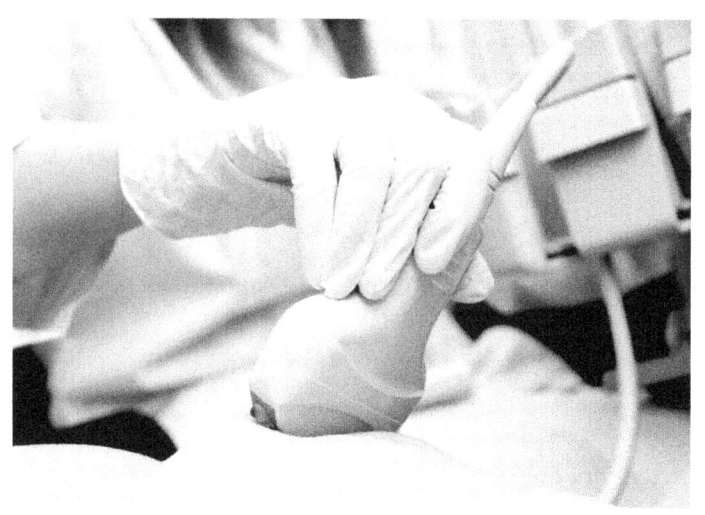

Mammograms

to·mo·SYN·the·sis
> A form of digital mammograms that creates a **3-D** picture of the breast using X-rays.

What

A regular mammogram typically takes two X-rays of each breast (one from top to bottom, and the other side to side). Digital tomosynthesis takes multiple X-ray pictures of each breast from many angles. The breast is positioned in a way similar to standard mammograms, but less pressure is applied. The X-ray tube moves in an arc around the breast while multiple images are take over approximately seven seconds. The information is then sent to a computer, where it is assembled to create clear 3D images of the breast. These multiple pictures create a layer-by-layer look at the breast tissue — one millimeter at a time — removing tissue overlap that may hide cancers or mistake dense breast tissue for cancer.

Why

Results with tomosynthesis are quite promising. Tomosynthesis can make breast cancers easier to see, especially in dense breast tissue, and may reduce the chances you will be called back for additional studies.

Better detection, fewer recalls

In one large study, researchers looked at data from 13 medical centers before and after they began using tomosynthesis. Digital mammograms with tomosynthesis detected one additional cancer for every 1,000 scans and resulted in 15% fewer false alarms – women called back for more tests and then found not to have cancer. The study was not designed to find out whether mammograms using tomosynthesis can save more lives than standard digital mammograms. The bottom line? Investigators found that the use of tomosynthesis ("3D") mammograms was associated with:

- Improved cancer detection rates, especially invasive cancers
- A decrease in call backs, which may lessen anxiety for patients

No access to tomosynthesis?

Dr. Robert Smith, American Cancer Society senior director of cancer screening, offers that the study described above does not mean all women should seek out 3-D mammograms. Although the study showed an important improvement in cancer detection rates, the improvement was small. The more dramatic finding, he observes, was having a lower chance of being called back for additional testing; that is, as compared to standard mammograms, tomosynthesis resulted in fewer false positives.

Step into the forest...

I love this analogy from *www.breastcancer.org:* Traditional mammograms take only one picture, across the entire breast, in two directions: Top to bottom and side to side. It's like standing on the edge of a forest, looking for a bird somewhere inside. To find the bird, it would be better to take 10 steps at a time through the forest and look all around you with each move. Welcome to the world of the 3-D mammogram, tomosynthesis. A radiologist analyzes the results of your exam and sends a report to your personal physician. For non-emergency situations, it usually takes a day or so to interpret, report, and deliver the results.

Did you know...

The Food and Drug Administration (FDA) approved breast tomosynthesis for use in February, 2011. By the following month, the Harvard Massachusetts General Hospital breast imaging team performed the first clinical breast tomosynthesis exam in the United States.

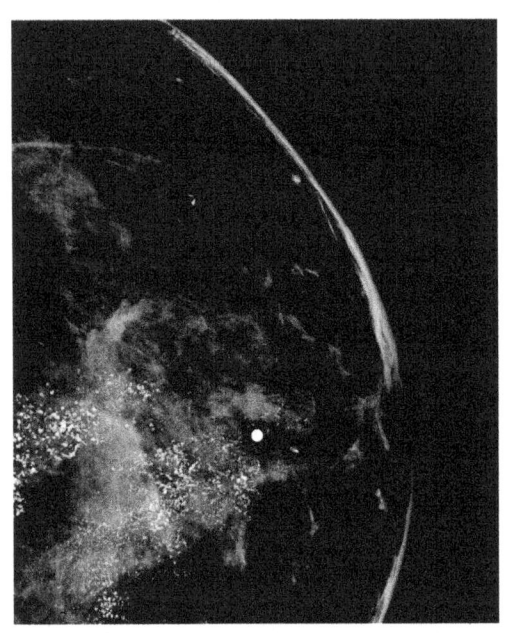

Mammogram
Malignant (cancer) calcifications

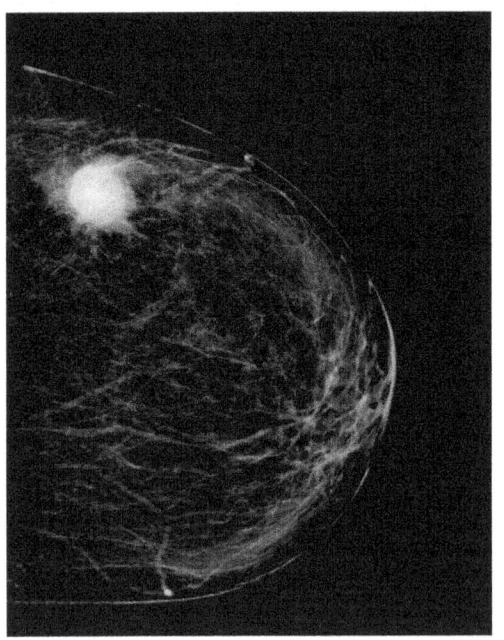

Mammogram
Mass (cancer)

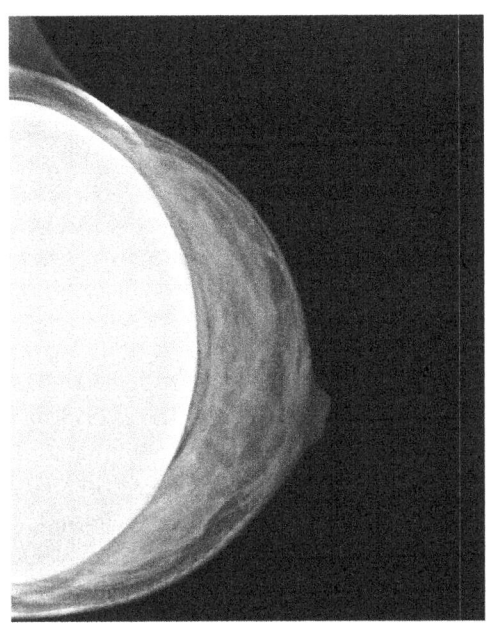

Mammogram
Implant obscures tissue

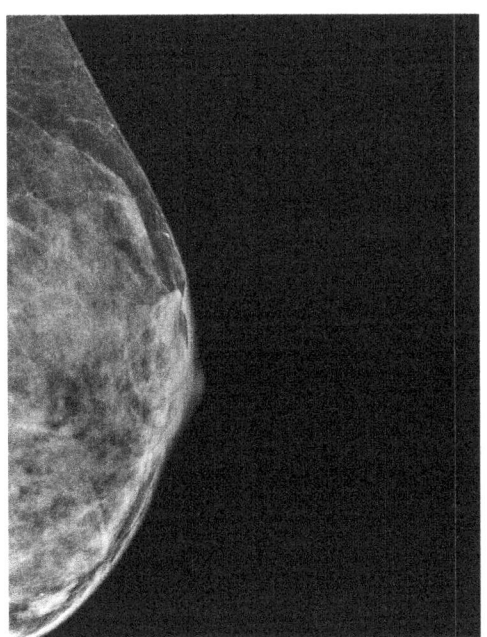

Mammogram
Cancer calcifications
Implant displacement (pushed away) view

Screen

screen·ing [skrēn´ ing]
Looking for cancer before a person has any symptoms.

Shared decision-making among patients and health care providers is critical to optimizing your care. Growing evidence points to not only a potential for over diagnosis with screening, but the fact that we may have underestimated the potential harms of screening individuals not at high risk for developing breast cancer. In this chapter, I will attempt to paint a picture that illustrates the trade-offs between potential benefits and harms of screening for breast cancer.

Benefits

Multiple clinical trials, involving over 600,000 women, have been conducted in the USA, Canada, the United Kingdom, and Sweden. The combined results point at a **reduction by one-fifth of the odds of dying of breast cancer**. Still, there have been numerous criticisms of the methods of the studies. Many patients in the studies "crossed over" to getting screened. On the other hand, might the reduction in breast cancer mortality actually be better with more modern imaging techniques?

Harms

Breast cancer screening can result in **false positive** results. A false positive is when the test says cancer may be present, when in fact it is not. We also have a risk of over diagnosis. Here, the test finds something that is clinically insignificant. Low-grade DCIS (ductal carcinoma *in situ*) may be an example. Unfortunately it is not always possible to distinguish cancers that are biologically insignificant from those that are potentially dangerous. Thus, we tend to treat all cancers.

Controversy

The odds of dying of cancer spread (metastasis) to distant sites are about one-third lower than they were in the 1980s. One model calculates that about half of this reduction is due to better systemic therapy such as chemotherapy and endocrine therapy; the other half is thought due to screening and local therapies.

Skip mammograms?

Screening tools are more likely to have value when they are applied to individuals at higher risk of developing cancer, and for whom early intervention is more effective than later treatment. So, how do we decide at what age a woman (at average risk for breast cancer) should begin mammograms?

Randomized trials show that mammograms reduce breast cancer mortality in those most likely to develop breast cancer. For those without a risk-raising genetic mutation such as BRCA (BReast CAncer gene), those under 40 are at low risk for breast cancer. **Risk starts to rise between 40 and 45, and rises more steeply for those between 45 and 65.** There are two groups of individuals for which mammograms would *not* likely provide value:

- Average-risk women under 40 years old
- Women with a limited life expectancy

Groups such as the American Cancer Society, the National Comprehensive Cancer Network (NCCN), and the US Preventative Task Force attempt to make screening recommendations by weighing potential benefits and potential harms (including unnecessary biopsies).

Shared decision-making

A care provider should help you make an informed, values-based decision about whether (and how often) to have screening for breast cancer. I hope that this chapter will help improve your knowledge about the pros and cons of screening, and to encourage you to take an active role in structuring your own breast cancer screening. First however, let's explore the screening tools.

Age

Screening benefits (including a reduction in breast cancer mortality) and harms (false positives and overdiagnosis) vary by age. For example, the ability of mammograms to detect cancer is higher among older women in general:

	Sensitivity
Early 40s	73%
Early 60s	85%

In addition, breast cancer incidence rises with age in general. Age and life expectancy therefore play an important role in determining mammogram efficacy. When should you begin getting mammograms?

- Under 40?

For women under 40 years who are at *average* risk of developing breast cancer, there is general consensus to *not* use screening mammograms. Not only is the risk of breast cancer lower for younger women, but mammogram performance is not as good as it is for older women: One study showed the recall rate (call-back for additional studies) was 13 percent for women ages 35 to 39, and the positive predictive value (the test says something is wrong, and the test is proven to be right at biopsy) was only about 1 percent.

- Over 40 years?

For women (at average risk) who are 40 years old or older, the expert guidelines are conflicting. Should you start screening at 40? 45? 50? We start with this fact: The numbers of lives saved by screening are lower for younger women than they are for older women. This is due, at least in part, to the fact that breast cancer incidence is lower among the younger group. In addition, the sensitivity (the disease is there, and the test finds it) and specificity (the disease is not there, and the test gets it right) is lower with younger women.

A meta-analysis (an analysis of a collection of studies) of eight randomized trials demonstrated a **15 percent relative reduction in breast cancer mortality** among women ages 39 to 48 who were randomized to have screening mammograms.

Let's look at age in a different way: How many women (at average risk for developing breast cancer) do we need to screen to prevent one woman from dying from the disease? Pooling the results of eight trials, the US Preventative Task Force estimates the following:

	Number Needed to Screen
Ages 30 to 49	1,904
Age 50 to 59	1,339

Age: When to stop mammograms

There is no general agreeement on the right age to stop having screening mammograms. It is not unreasonable to continue screening if you have a life expectancy of at least 10 years, irrespective of your age. Screening mammograms can lead to earlier stage presentations, but may not meaningfully improve your survival odds. Why? If you are older, you have competing risks such as heart attack and stroke. In addition, screening mammograms may find breast disease (such as low-grade ductal carcinoma *in situ* or DCIS) that is not clinically meaningful.

Unfortunately, none of the 8 randomized trials included women 75 and older. Observational studies suggest a *possible* decrease in breast cancer mortality among healthy women 80 and older who are regularly screened with mammography; however, these studies are limited by various biases (lead time, length time, and selection types).

Mammogram frequency uncertainty

We have limited data on the optimal frequency for having screening mammograms. Some advocate for yearly mammograms, while others suggest screening every two years. Here are some research findings from the Breast Cancer Surveillance Consortium:

- **Premenopausal women** who had every two year screening had *less* favorable cancers (Stage IIB and higher).
- **Women using menopausal hormones** who had every two year screening had *less* favorable cancers.
- **Postmenopausal women not on hormones** did equally well with screening mammograms annually or every two years.

Harms in more detail

While mammograms reduce the chances of dying of breast cancer, there are some potential harms associated with screening:

- Insignificant cancers

  Diagnosis of cancers that would otherwise never have caused symptoms or death can expose you to immediate risks (surgical deformity or toxicities from radiation therapy, hormone therapy, or chemotherapy), late side effects (e.g. arm swelling). Although management is tailored to individual tumor characteristics, there is no reliable way to distinguish which cancer would never progress in an individual patient; therefore, some treatment is nearly always recommended. Incidence studies in the United States found that at least 20% of screen-detected breast cancers are over diagnosed.

- False-Positives

  About 10 percent of women will be recalled from each screening examination for further testing, and only 5 percent called back will have cancer. These extra tests have not only financial costs, but can cause anxiety as well. A higher chance of a false positive result occurs among younger women, those who have had previous biopsies of the breast, patients with a positive family history of breast cancer, estrogen use, an increased time interval between screenings, no comparison of the current mammogram with previous ones, and a radiologist's personal tendency to call mammograms abnormal.

Mammograms: Potential Harms (ccontinued)

- Mammogram-Induced Breast Cancer

The breast dose associated with a typical two-view mammogram is approximately 4 mSv (milli-Sieverts). Latency is at least 8 years, and the increased risk is life-long. In theory, annual mammograms in women aged 40 to 80 years may cause up to one breast cancer per 1,162 women. The reduction in death thanks to screening mammograms greatly outweigh the risk of death due to radiation-induced cancers.

As medical questions often have no clear-cut answers, transparent information is critical to your decision making. In this context, I present a fact box developed at the Harding Center for Risk Literacy. In the table, the numbers refer to 1,000 women over 50 years of age who participated in screening for 10 years or more (screening group), compared to 1,000 women of the same age who did not participate in screening during the same time period (control group).

Breast Cancer Early Detection by Mammography

For women 50 years or older who did or did not participate in screening for about 10 years (results for every 1,000 women)

	No Screening	Screening
Benefits		
How many **died from breast cancer**?	5	4
How many died from all types of cancer?	21	21
Harms		
How many had false alarms or biopsies	-	100
How many with non-progressive cancer had unnecessary partial or complete breast removal?	-	5

Risk

Many factors determine a woman's risk of breast cancer. Some are genetic and relate to family history, others are based on personal factors such as reproductive and medical history. We have several tools to calculate your personal risk of developing breast cancer. Although these tools can estimate your risk, they cannot tell whether or not you will get breast cancer.

Gail model

The most commonly used tool to calculate breast cancer risk is the Breast Cancer Risk Assessment Tool, also known as the Gail Model tool. This simple tool incorporates variables such as age, race, history of breast disease, age at onset of menses, family history, and number of full-term pregnancies. It calculates a woman's risk of developing breast cancer within the next five years, and within her lifetime (up to age 90). You can find this easy-to-use tool here:

Limitations

The Gail Tool does *not* give a good estimate of risk in some women including those with:

- A personal history of invasive breast cancer, ductal carcinoma *in situ* (DCIS) or lobular carcinoma *in situ* (LCIS);
- A strong family history of breast cancer, who may have an inherited gene mutation (such as BRCA1);
- The original model was based on data from white women. It has been updated to estimate risk for African-American women, Asian-Ameri can and Pacific Islander women. However, it's still not clear how well the model works in other racial/ethnic groups.

Other tools use family history to estimate breast cancer risk. These include BRCAPRO, IBIS (which uses the Tyrer-Cuzik model) and BOADICEA. Such tools can be particularly useful for women with one or more relatives with breast or ovarian cancer.

SCREENING MAMMOGRAMS
NUMBER TO PREVENT ONE BREAST CANCER DEATH

Age	False positive	Need biopsy	DCIS or invasive cancer	Number needed to be screened
40-49	98	9	3	**1,904**
50-59	87	11	5	**1,339**
60-69	79	12	7	377
70-79	69	12	8	?
80-89	59	11	2	?

* estimates are for a single screening for a woman at *average* risk

Exam

Clinical breast examination (CBE)
CBE by a healthcare provider has not been tested independently; it was used in conjunction with mammography in one Canadian trial, and was the comparator modality versus mammography in another trial. It would be challenging to assess the value of CBE as a screening modality when it is used alone versus usual care (no screening activity).

And there are potential harms: In the community, the false-positive rate is 1% to 12%. In addition, there can be so-called false negative results, leading to potential false reassurance and delay to cancer diagnosis. In fact, of women with cancer, up to approximately 40% will have a clear CBE. Sensitivity (the exam finds cancer when it is there) increases over time.

Breast self-exam
Breast self-exam (BSE) has been compared with no screening activity, and has *not* been shown to reduce breast cancer mortality. There have been two large, randomized trials (China; Russia) examining BSE. Neither showed improvements in outcomes among those that performed regular breast self-examinations:

- *Shanghai:* From 1989 through 1991, 266,064 women associated with 519 factories in Shanghai were randomly assigned to a breast self-exam instruction or not. Initial instruction in BSE was followed by reinforcement sessions 1 and 3 years later, BSE under medical supervision at least every 6 months for 5 years, and by ongoing reminders to practice BSE monthly. The women were followed through December 2000. Intensive instruction in BSE did *not* reduce mortality from breast cancer.

- *St. Petersburg:* No benefit to breast self-examination.

Limitations
Breast self-exam has potential harms: In the Chinese study, the biopsy rate was 1.8% among the study population (compared with 1% in the control group), with no improvement in cancer detection with screening. Still, in countries where regular imaging is not done, breast exams (by you and a medical professional) seem reasonable.

Screening: Emerging tools

Ultrasound

Many tools for the early detection of breast cancer are under investigation. Some are already used in diagnosis and staging, and are widely available. But should we use ultrasound for *routine* screening? Mammograms combined with breast ultrasound may find slightly more breast cancers than mammograms alone for women with *dense* breasts. However, mammography plus breast ultrasound leads to more false positive results than mammography alone. Ultrasound is not currently used routinely for screening among women at average risk for breast cancer. If you don't have access to 3D mammograms, and you have dense breast issue, an elevated cancer risk, or implants, adding screening ultrasound to a regular screening mammogram can improve cancer detection.

Tomosynthesis (3D) mammograms

Computer software combines multiple 2D X-ray images to create a three-dimensional (3D) image. Radiologists must have special training to read these 3D images. Combining 2D mammography with breast tomosynthesis can increase the odds of finding breast cancer, particularly if you have dense breasts and/or are still menstruating. Tomosynthesis can also lower the "call-back" rate.

Nuclear medicine breast imaging

Nuclear medicine breast imaging (or molecular breast imaging) uses short-lived radioactive agents given through an IV. These agents are absorbed into tissues, including the breast. Breast cancer cells absorb more of the agents than do healthy cells, and cancer cells can then be imaged with a special camera. Nuclear medicine breast imaging is under study for use in breast cancer screening, diagnosis and staging.

Examples include breast-specific gamma imaging (BSGI) and positron emission mammography (PEM). The radioactive agents used in BSGI emit gamma rays that are tracked by a special camera. For the PEM, radioactive sugar is injected. Cancer cells tend to consume more sugar than normal cells and this can help find tumors. Unfortunately, a dose of radiation that is 15 to 20 times higher than the dose from a mammogram is given.

Thermography

Thermography (digital infrared imaging devices) uses infrared light to measure temperature differences on the breast surface. Breast cancer can cause abnormal heat patterns that can theorectically be detected. However, there is no solid scientific evidence that thermography measures of heat can help find breast cancers. We have no randomized controlled trials evaluating its impact on early detection or mortality.

 Thermography is FDA-approved for the detection of breast cancer, but is not approved as a sole screeng tool for screening. It's approved to be used in conjunction with mammography. The FDA warnes that **thermography should not be used as an alternative to mammograms** for breast cancer screening or diagnosis, in a safety communication issued February 25, 2019;

Breast MRI for women with dense breast tissue

Breast magnetic resonance imaging (MRI) uses magnetic fields to create a breast image. There is no ionizing radiation. It is more invasive than mammograms, as MRI requires a contrast agent that is given through an IV before the scan. Breast MRI is mostly used for breast cancer diagnosis and staging for select individuals. It is also used in breast cancer screening for women at higher risk.

MRI evaluates the blood flow pattern through the breast tissues, looking for areas where blood rapidly pools and then washes away; this occurs at cancer sites because of angiogenesis, or the formation of new blood vessels, as directed by the cancer itself.

Mammography plus breast MRI is under investigation for screening average-risk women with dense breast tissue: MRI does not care about your breast density, so it can outperform mammograms and ultrasound. If you have very dense breasts, you may want to ask your health care provider about adding MRI to mammogram screening. Alas, breast MRI is associated with a relatively high chance of a false positive (the test indicates that cancer is present, when in reality it is not; this leads to additional tudies and biopsies), is expensive, and not a particularly enjoyable experienve (you need to lie face down in what can be a claustrophobia-inducing tube, with clanging noises ringing out).

Screening: High-risk

Experts use your personal and family medical histories, genetic tests, lifestyle and exposures, and other factors to assess risk and make recommendations for breast screening and risk management. If you are at higher risk of breast cancer, you may need to be screened earlier, more often, and with additional imaging tools than women at average risk. Let's examine some factors that may place you in the high-risk category.

There are inherited genetic conditions that can markedly raise your risk for developing breast cancer. These include having a breast cancer gene mutation (BRCA1 or BRCA2), or a first-degree relative with such a mutation. Having a strong family history of breast cancer (for example, your mother and/or sister) developing at age 45 or younger can markedly increase your risk. Li-Fraumeni, Cowden, and Bannayan-Riley-Ruvalcaba syndromes are associated with genetic changes that can put you in the high risk category. This holds true if you or a first-degree relative has one of these syndromes, or a p53 or PTEN gene mutation.

A personal history of invasive breast cancer or ductal carcinoma *in situ* (DCIS) can also raise your risk significantly, as can a personal hisory of lobular carcinoma *in situ* (LCIS) or atypical hyperplasia (atypical ductal hyperplasia (ADH) or atypical lobular hyperplasia (ALH)). Finally, a personal history of radiation treatment to the chest region (especially if this occurred before the age of 30) puts you into the high-risk for breast cancer category. To understand your breast cancer risk and the actions you can take to manage it, please consult with medical experts who have advanced training in risk assessment and cancer genetics.

Is there a role for MRI in breast cancer screening?

MRI can improve cancer detection, but increases callback and biopsy rates (which can increase anxiety levels). Those with a lifetime breast cancer risk of over 20% should consider combining MRI and mammography. The current American Cancer Society recommendations for breast MRI screening don't address the timing of MRI in conjunction with mammograms.

RISK GROUPS

High-risk 30%+	• BRCA mutation • Other hereditary cancer syndromes (for example, Li-Fraumeni Syndrome; Cowden Syndrome)
Intermediate risk 20-29%	• Breast biopsy shows *atypical* hyperplasia, or lobular carcinoma *in situ* (LCIS) • A calculated risk of 20% to 29% based on family history, personal health history, or certain genetic markers
Average risk 10-13%	• None of the above factors

The timing of screening MRIs to optimize performance is controversial. The American College of Radiology offers that premenopausal women should have their breast screening MRI scheduled between days 7 and 14 after the first day of their menstrual cycle; however, data supporting this recommendation are sparse. One study of screening MRIs in 244 premenopausal women found that the menstrual cycle phase did *not* significantly impact MRI performance.

Not everyone can have an MRI
Some conditions may make you a poor candidate for an MRI. These include: 1) pregnancy; 2) an allergy to gadolinium-based contrast; 3) having certain implanted devices (for example, pacemakers); 4) your kidney function is inadequate; and 5) you have uncontrolled anxiety or claustrophobia.

MRI and mammogram

Mammograms use very low doses of radiation to make X-ray images of the breast. X-rays do not penetrate dense breast tissue very well, making mammography more challenging. Compared with mammograms, MRI is more sensitive in finding abnormalities within the breasts. MRI scans use radio waves and strong magnets instead of X-rays. The radio wave energy is absorbed and then released in a pattern determined by the type of tissue. A computer then translates this pattern into a highly detailed image. For a breast MRI, a contrast liquid known as gadolinium is injected into a vein before or during the scan to allow better visualization of the details.

For the MRI, you lie inside a narrow tube with your face down on a platform designed for the procedure. This platform has openings for each breast. This allows for imaging without compressing the breasts. You have to stay still for the imaging procedure.

Several large, prospective, non-randomized studies have examined the efficacy of adding breast screening MRIs to annual mammograms for women at high risk of developing breast cancer. These studies included women with BRCA gene mutations or a strong family history of breast cancer. Despite differences in patient population and in MRI technique, all of these studies showed MRI to be more sensitive at detecting breast cancer compared with mammograms.

Limitations

While MRI can detect smaller tumors than can mammograms, MRI has important limitations: Call-back rates are higher for MRI, ranging from 8% to 17% for imaging and 3% to 15% for biopsy. Subsequent rounds of screening typically have lower call-back rates.

Risk Management Guidelines

The National Comprehensive Cancer Network (NCCN) is a consortium of cancer centers with experts in management of hereditary cancer. The NCCN updates their guidelines for risk management for people with hereditary risk for cancer, based on the latest research. In general, NCCN guidelines dictate the standard of care for high-risk patients.

Early detection

Regular screening tests (along with appropriate health management) can reduce your chance of dying from breast cancer. Screening tests can find breast cancer early, when the chances of survival are highest. Here are some elements of a personal action plan:

- *Watch for symptoms*

  Breast cancer warning signs vary among women. If you are unsure about a concerning finding, it is best to see a healthcare provider. Common symptoms include a change in the look or feel of your breast or nipple, or a nipple discharge.

- *Know your breasts*

  Breast self-exam (BSE) seemed promising when first introduced. However, studies on its effectiveness at finding breast cancer early and improving survival suggest it may not offer the same benefits as other screening tests such as a clinical breast exam (by a health provider), mammogram or a breast MRI (for those at higher risk of getting breast cancer).

- *Know screening recommendations*

  Breast cancer screening can help find breast cancer early, when the chances of survival are highest. Women at higher risk may need breast cancer screening earlier and more often than other women. Breast cancer screening is not recommended for most men.

Next, we'll turn to abnormal findings on imaging or physical exam.

MRI AND SCREENING

	Holland	Canada	UK	Germany	USA
Sensitivity (%)*					
MRI	80	77	77	91	100
Mammograms	33	36	40	33	25
Ultrasound	N/A	33	N/A	40	N/A
Specificity (%)					
MRI	90	95	81	97	95
Mammograms	95	>99	93	97	98
Ultrasound	N/A	96	N/A	91	N/A

N/A = not applicable

* **Sensitivity** (true positive rate) measures the percentage of cancers that are correctly identified.

****Specificity** (true negative rate) measures the percentage of healthy people who are correctly identified as *not* having breast cancer).

If you have an abnormal mammogram or a concerning physical finding,

what's next? Follow-up typically begins with less invasive tests such as *diagnostic* mammograms or breast ultrasound. The radiologist examines the images to determine whether the abnormal finding looks suspicious:

- *Not suspicious-appearing*

If the lesion clearly doesn't look like cancer on imaging, you may not need any more testing. An example is a simple cyst.

- *Suspicious-appearing*

Typically, a biopsy (a tissue sampling, often using a needle) is done, and the abnormal tissue then sent to a pathologist to examine it for cancer.

Most calcifications seen on mammograms are *not* cancer. However, calcifications are sometimes a sign of cancer. We may conveniently classify calcifications into one of 3 categories:

1) Benign (top photo on left)
2) Intermediate concern
3) Higher probability of cancer (bottom photo on left)

Benign calcifications are typically larger, coarser, and round with smooth margins. They may be scattered or diffuse. Malignant calcifications are typically grouped or clustered, pleomorphic (varying in size and shape), fine and with linear branching.

Mammogram: Screening versus Diagnostic

Screening mammograms are used for individuals with no symptoms or signs of breast cancer. Screening mammograms try to find breast cancer when it is too small to be felt by you or your care provider. Diagnostic mammograms are used for individuals with a known breast problem. Examples include a lump or nipple discharge, or an abnormal area found in a screening mammogram. We sometimes use diagnostic mammograms for patients without breast problems who were previously treated for breast cancer. During a diagnostic mammogram, the images are reviewed by the radiologist while you are there, so that more images may be obtained if needed to look at a concerning area.

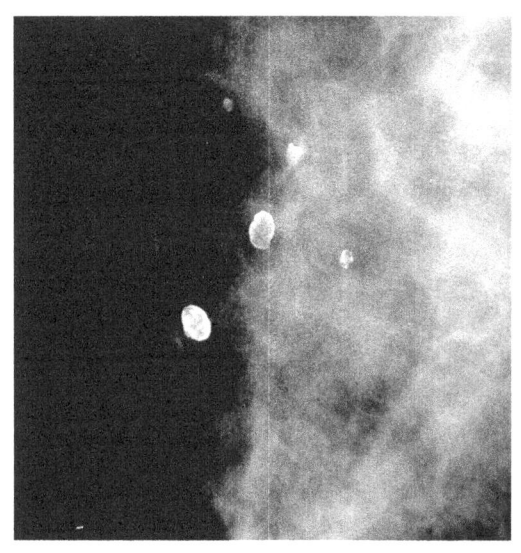

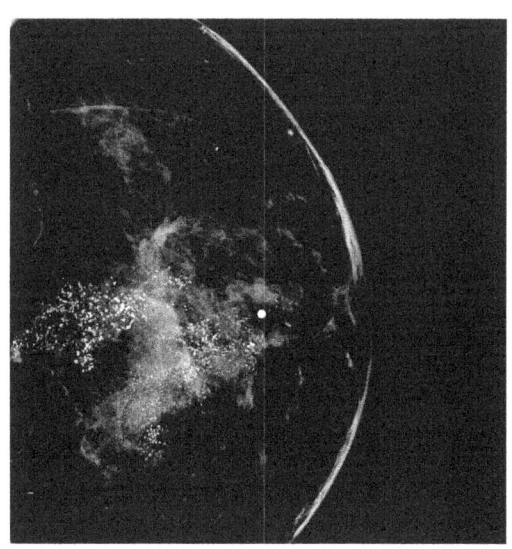

Diagnostic mammograms

Sometimes, special images known as spot (or magnification) views are taken, in order to make a small area of concern easier to evaluate. Diagnostic mammograms may be interpreted in one of 3 ways:

- **Not cancer:** An area that looked abnormal on a screening mammogram appears normal. You typically then return to routine annual mammograms.

- **Probably not cancer:** An area that looked abnormal on a screening mammogram is probably not cancer, but it is common to be asked to come back in 4 to 6 months to re-check.

- **Looks like may be cancer:** A biopsy is recommended.

Special case: Women under 30 with symptoms

For women under 30, most breast lumps are benign (not cancer). A first step is a clinical breast exam (CBE), a physical exam performed by a skilled health care provider. The clinician should carefully feel your breasts and underarm area for any changes abnormalities (such as a lump). Examples of abnormal findings that may be discovered on clinical exam include:

- A dominant lump in the breast or underarm area
- Change in breast size or shape
- Dimpling or puckering of skin
- Pulling in of the nipple or other breast parts
- Nipple discharge
- Pain
- Swelling, redness, warmth, or darkening of the breast

Additional evaluation may include a breast ultrasound (and for selected women, a mammogram). Selected women may require a biopsy to determine whether a lump is breast cancer or not.

MAMMOGRAMS

BI-RADS Category	
1 Negative	No significant abnormality.
2 Benign	No sign of cancer, but the reporting radiologist chooses to describe a finding thought benign (e.g. benign calcifications).
3 Probably benign	98% chance *not* cancer. May be suggested to repeat imaging in 6 months, and regularly thereafter to ensure stability.
4 Suspicious	Findings do not definitely look like cancer, but could be. Radiologist concerned enough to recommend a biopsy.
5 Highly suggestive of cancer	High chance (over 95%) cancer present. Biopsy is strongly recommended.
6 Known cancer	May be used to assess response to treatment.

* We use a standard system to describe mammogram findings and results. This system (called the Breast Imaging Reporting and Data System or BI-RADS) sorts results into categories as above. By categorizing in this way, we can describe the mammogram findings using the common terminology. This makes accurately communicating about test results (and recommended) much easier.

DCIS

Now that we are in the mammogram screening era, there are no specific symptoms (or findings on physical exam) for the vast majority of individuals with ductal carcinoma *in situ*. Prior to the use of widespread screening mammograms, DCIS would present as a mass that could be felt, nipple discharge, or scaly skin of (and around) the nipple. Let's look at the more modern age:

Mammograms

Approximately ninety percent of woman with DCIS have suspicious microcalcifications on mammograms. Looked at differently, DCIS represents 80 percent of all breast cancers presenting with calcifications. Less commonly, patients with DCIS may present with a mass or other change in the soft tissue of the breast.

If you care team suspects that you may have DCIS, diagnostic mammograms of both breasts should be performed. The radiologist reading your mammogram looks for particular patterns of microcalcifications that highly suggest DCIS may be present.

Linear branching calcifications, or ones that have several different shapes (pleomorphic) are more commonly associated with DCIS that is more aggressive (high nuclear grade, so-called comedonecrosis), while more fine, granular calcifications are more likely to be associated with a lower grade DCIS. Finally, sometimes there will be clusters of calcifications that are scattered focally (multifocal) or throughout the breast (multicentric).

MRI

Magnetic resonance imaging (MRI) is *not* routinely performed as a part of DCIS evaluation, at least in many centers of excellence: We do not fully understand it optimal use for DCIS. For some, it may healp determine the extend of DCIS, but I am unaware of high level evidence suggesting that it improves longer term outcomes.

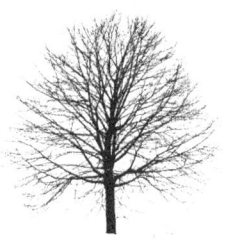

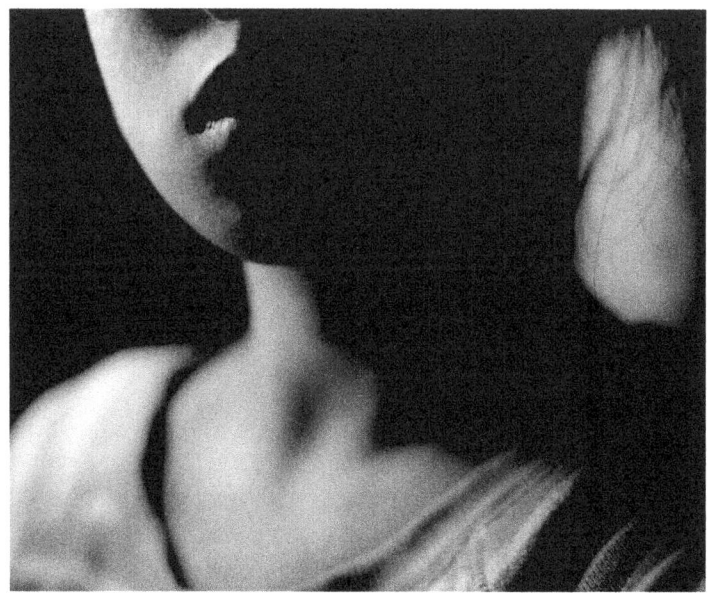

Breast density

Breast density may be reported on your mammogram report, but is often subjective. In addition to a BI-RADS system describing our level of suspicion (see table to the right), the BI-RADS system also classifies breast density:

- *Almost entirely fatty*
Because fatty breasts have little fibrous and glandular tissue, the mammogram would likely be able to see anything abnormal.

- *Having scattered fibroglandular density*
There are a few areas of fibrous and glandular tissue in the breast.

- *Heterogeneously dense*
The breast has more areas of fibrous and glandular tissue throughout the breast. This can make finding small masses more challenging.

- *Extremely dense*
The breast has a lot of fibrous and glandular tissue. This can make it harder to see a cancer, as it can blend in with normal tissues (like finding a snowball in a snow field).

Dense breasts have a significantly higher risk of developing breast cancer. But does the presence of dense breasts among those with breast cancer affect the risk of dying of the disease? To examine the relationship between breast density and breast cancer mortality, researchers analyzed data from the Breast Cancer Surveillance Consortium (BCSC), a population-based registry of breast imaging facilities in the USA. They limited data collection to the five BCSC registries that consistently collect data on body mass index (BMI), in order to be able to adjust for such factors.

After adjusting for other health factors, the analysis showed that the overall group of patients with high-density breasts did not have a higher risk of death from breast cancer, as compared with patients with lower density breasts. However, subgroup analysis suggested that there might be an increased risk of breast cancer death among women with low density (BI-RADS 1) who were either obese (2-times increase in risk) or had primary cancers measuring 2 cm or greater (1.55-times increase in risk).

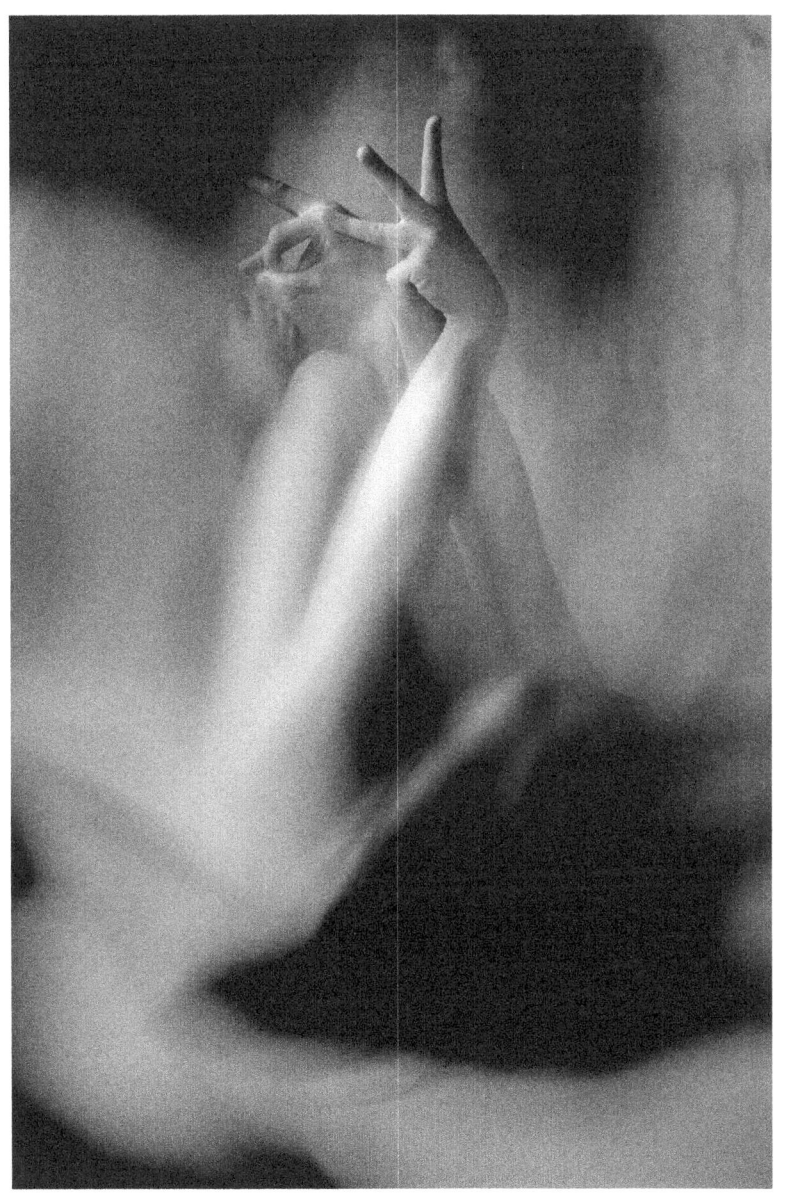

BIOPSY

Biopsy types

An outpatient biopsy using a needle is usually a fairly simple procedure, and is generally preferred to a surgical biopsy. Too often, surgical biopsies are performed on women who have abnormal mammograms, rather than the much safer and less invasive needle biopsy. In the USA, about 20% of biopsies turn out to be cancer. In countries such as Sweden (where only the most suspicious lesions have a biopsy), about 80% turn out to be cancerous (malignant).

Least invasive

A needle biopsy uses a hollow needle to remove samples of tissue or cells from the breast. The material is then sent to a pathologist, who studies these samples under a microscope to see if they contain cancer or other concerning findings. There are two types of needle biopsies:

- **Core needle biopsy**

    A core biopsy may be used to investigate a lump that can be felt in the breast. It may also be used to assess a lesion that cannot be felt, but is visible on imaging. A core needle biopsy can be quite accurate and is less invasive than surgery. Core needle biopsy removes a narrow cylinder of tissue. While there is a small chance of bruising or infection, it is generally accurate, and (if a cancer is present) can provide information about the cancer type, grade (aggressiveness), and receptor status (Is the cancer driven by estrogen? Progesterone? HER2?)

- **Fine needle aspiration (FNA)**

    FNA removes cells from a suspicious lump, and is only used for lumps that can be felt. The needle used is thinner than ones used for core needle biopsies. While core needle biopsy is often the first choice for palpable masses, FNA is sometimes done as a quick means of sampling a breast lump felt during a clinical breast exam or a concerning underarm (axillary) lymph node. The false positive rate is about 1 to 2%. The false negative rate can be on the order of 40%, so if the FNA does not show cancer, your care team may recommend the obtaining of more tissue (depending on what the FNA demonstrates).

Most invasive

Most health care providers will first try to figure out the cause of a breast abnormality by doing a needle biopsy. Less commonly, a surgical biopsy is needed. A surgical (or open) biopsy is done by cutting the breast to take out all or part of the lump so it can be looked at under a microscope. The vast majority of open breast biopsies are performed with either local anesthesia alone or local anesthesia combined with intravenous sedation. General anesthesia is tyically used for more complex situations; for example, it may be employed when multiple abnormalities must be removed and local anesthesia would be insufficient.

Incisional biopsy

A incisional biopsy removes only part (but more than does a needle biopsy) of the suspicious area, enough to make a diagnosis. It is only done if the tumor is too big to be removed with an excisional biopsy. Incisional biopsies are not commonly performed.

Excisional biopsy (lumpectomy)

An excisional biopsy removes the entire abnormality in the breast. It is typically done by a surgeon in an operating room (OR). Your surgeon will use local anesthetia to numb the area that will be sampled. You will also need sedation via an intravenous line. Typically, the procedure is an outpatient one: Most individuals do not have to stay in the hospital overnight.

Before surgery, a wire-localization or needle-localization procedure is often performed, if the abnormal area in the breast cannot be felt. A radiologist uses mammograms, ultrasound, or other imaging to guide a very thin wire into the suspicious area of the breast. The surgeon can then use this wire to find the area of concern during your surgery.

In the operating room, the breast tissue that is removed is usually X-rayed. This lets the surgeon and radiologist match the suspicious areas on the mammogram with those in the biopsy tissue to ensure the correct tissue was removed. If the areas do not match, the surgeon may try again to remove the correct tissue or may wait to do another biopsy.

Excisional biopsy (continued)

The incision should be long enough to provide adequate exposure and to ensure that the mass can be removed as a single specimen with a small margin of grossly normal tissue. The surgeon should orient the specimen, and the pathologist should ink all margins. Although the goal of an excisional biopsy is to diagnose cancer, sometimes the surgeon may be able to fully remove the cancer. In these cases, excisional biopsy may be the only breast surgery needed to treat the cancer. For others, lymph nodes may also need to be removed (in a second surgery at a later date).

Results

After tissue is removed, the material is sent to a doctor known as a **pathologist.** The pathologist examines the tissue, including with the use of a microscope and determines whether the tissue contains cancer. A pathology report (including the diagnosis) is issued, and sent to the ordering physician. The report may have material added at a later date, so there can be more than one report for a single biopsy session.

Your pathology report provides your diagnosis. Most of the initial information comes within 7 to 10 days after your surgery, and you will usually have all the results within a few weeks. Your doctor can let you know when the results come in. If you don't hear from your doctor, call the office. A physician (such as your radiologist, surgeon or your oncologist) will review the main findings of the report and answer any questions you may have. The report itself is prepared for healthcare providers, making the language sometimes confusing for the patient. Still, understanding the basic parts of the report can help you to be a better consumer. Because each individual's breast cancer is unique, it's important to understand the underlying biology of your cancer in order to personalize your management plan.

 Ask for a copy of your pathology report for your personal records.

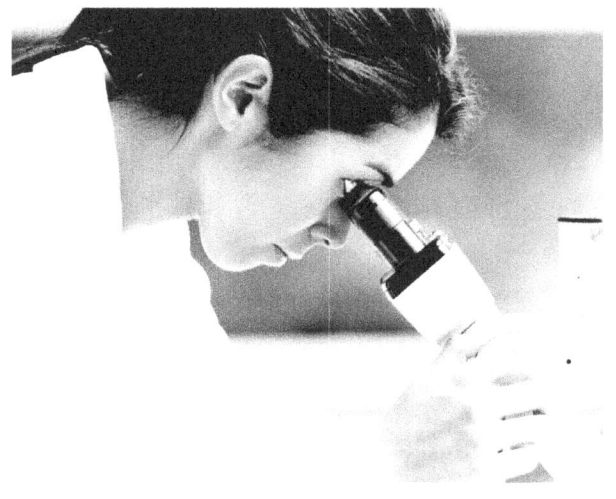

1. **Pathologist** receives biopsy material.

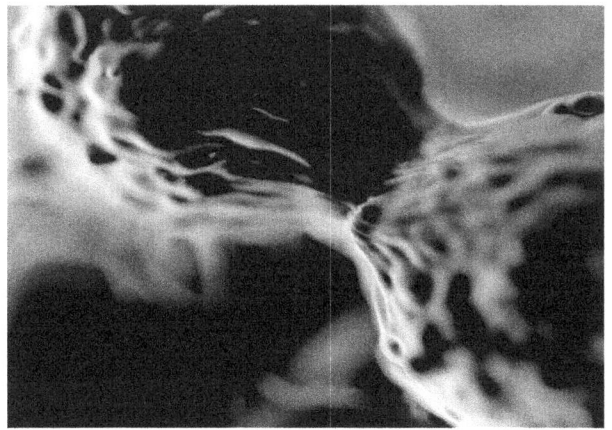

2. Tissue examined under a microscope.

Basics

Cancer is a condition in which cells do not die at the normal rate. As the cell growth exceeds cell death, a mass of tissue (tumor) can form. Breast cancer happens when cells in the breast divide and grow abnormally. Many (but not all) breast cancers grow slowly and are not detected until 10 to 15 years before we can detect it. Up to 75% of breast cancers begin in the milk ducts, while 10 to 15% begin in the lobules. The remainder start in other breast tissues. **Benign** means not cancer.

Non-invasive or invasive?

We may conveniently divide breast cancer into two categories: Invasive versus non-invasive breast cancer. The latter is also referred to as ductal carcinoma *in situ* (DUK-tul kar-sin-O-ma in SY-too), or DCIS. Only about 20 to 25% of breast cancer is non-invasive, with the rest being invasive.

- Ductal carcinoma *in situ* (DCIS)

   Abnormal cells are confined to the milk ducts. *In situ* means "remaining in place." With DCIS, the cancer cells are contained within the milk ducts; there is no invasion through the breast duct walls into surrounding tissue (stroma). Many clinicians believe we should not think of DCIS as a true cancer (as it cannot spread in its pure form), but the classification has not yet changed.

   Please note that lobular carcinoma *in situ* (LCIS) is not a cancer, but can raise the future risk of getting a cancer in either breast.

Biopsies are performed to make the diagnosis. If you are found to have ductal carcinoma *in situ*, more surgery is typically performed to make sure that all of the DCIS is removed, ideally with a cancer-free zone (clear margins) around the removed DCIS. For some women, this means a lumpectomy; for others, it may mean breast removal (for example if the DCIS is widespread throughout the breast). In the next chapter, we will look more closely at DCIS, and as well as some non-cancer findings.

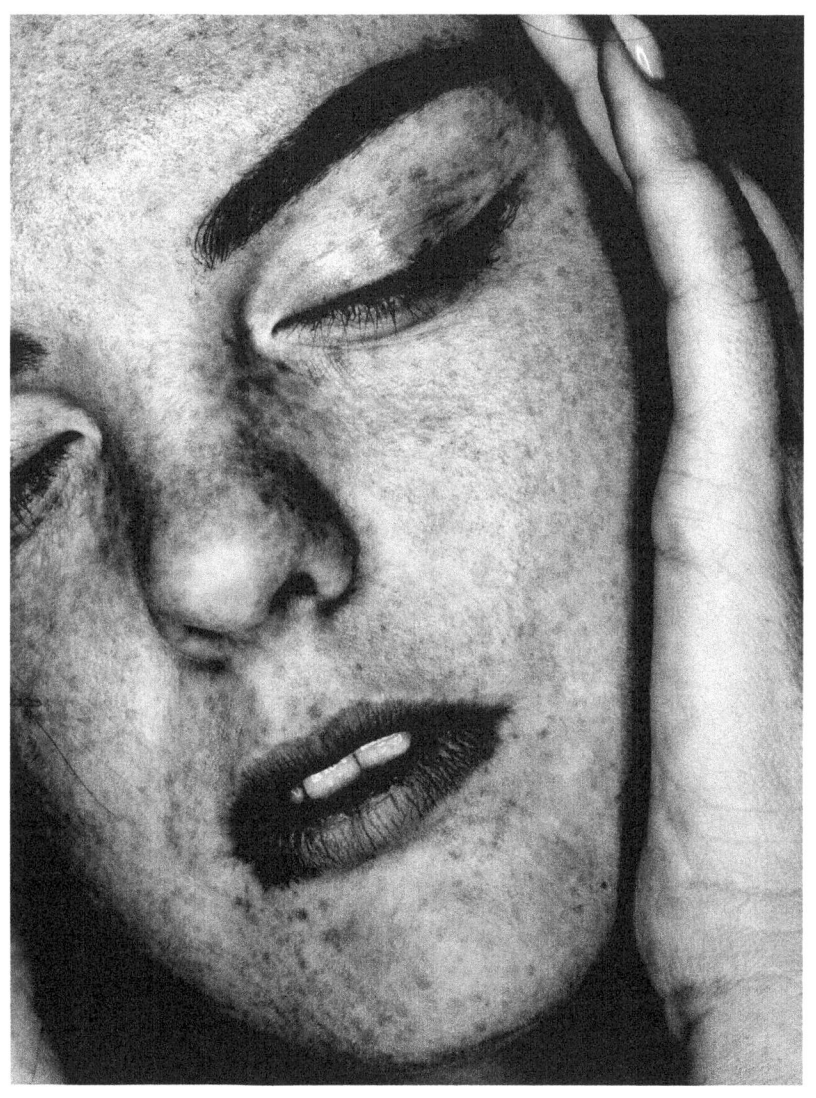

PATHOLOGY

UNDER THE MICROSCOPE

DCIS (ductal carcinoma in situ)

Biopsy

After a breast biopsy or surgery, the removed tissue is sent to a pathologist, a medical doctor who specializes in the examination of such specimens. They examine the cells and tissue grossly, and then under a microscope. The pathologist's observations and thoughts are then provided in your pathology report. Typically, this report is issued no sooner than several days after the pathologist receives the tissue. The information in the pathology report is critical to optimizing your management.

Basics

It's *not* really a cancer: **Ductal carcinoma* in situ (DCIS) is not breast cancer as many commonly understood it.** Non-invasive "cancers" stay within the milk ducts or milk lobules in the breast: The abnormal cells in DCIS have not spread outside the milk ducts (*in situ* means "remaining in place") into other parts of the breast, or to other parts of the body. In its pure form, DCIS is non-lethal because it stays in its normal place. However, DCIS is very important because it is the immediate precursor of invasive breast cancers, which are potentially deadly. Without treatment, DCIS may develop into an invasive breast cancer (which can then potentially spread to regional nodes, or even metastasize to distant parts of the body such as the bones, lungs, liver, or other sites).

Ductal carcinoma *in situ* encompasses a wide spectrum of diseases ranging from low-grade lesions that are not life-threatening to high-grade lesions that may hide bits of invasive breast cancer within. DCIS is characterized by the growth of abnormal cells that are bounded by the basement membrane of the breast ducts. DCIS is also called intraductal (within the milk ducts) carcinoma. You may also hear the terms "pre-invasive" or "pre-cancerous" to describe it.

---

* Cancer that arises in epithelial cells. Epithelial tissues line the outer surfaces of organs and blood vessels throughout the body, as well as the inner surfaces of cavities in many internal organs.

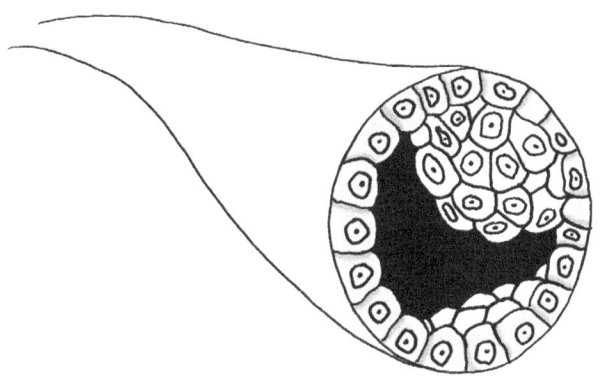

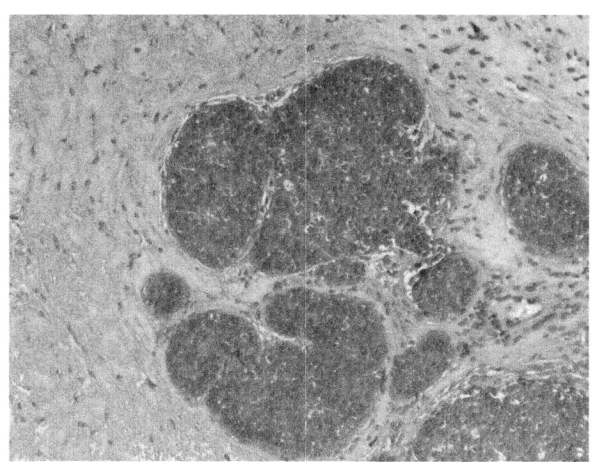

DCIS
Abnormal cells are contained in the milk ducts. In situ ("remaining in its original place") means the cells have not left the milk ducts to invade nearby breast tissue.

DCIS

Prior to widespread screening mammograms, clinicians usually diagnosed ductal carcinoma *in situ* (DCIS or intraductal carcinoma) by surgically removing a suspicious breast mass. While first described in 1893, DCIS was rarely diagnosed before the 1980s. Today a quarter of breast cancers diagnosed in the USA are DCIS, a non-invasive breast cancer.

The recognition of DCIS as a specific disease distinct from invasive breast cancer occurred gradually, primarily during the first half of the 20th century. It was rare during that time, accounting for only 1%–2% of newly diagnosed breast cancers, and was usually detected when it formed a large palpable mass. Mastectomy became the standard therapy, and it typically cured the rare patient who presented with DCIS. With the rise of screening mammograms at the tail end of the 20th century, radiologist had the tools to catch this early stage breast cancer. Ductal carcinoma *in situ* sometimes produces calcium deposits in the ducts, and it is this mammogram-detected calcium (rather than a mass) that leads to the diagnosis of DCIS for up to 1 in 4 patients with DCIS.

Currently, we believe that invasive breast cancer evolves through a non-obligatory series of increasingly abnormal "stages" over long periods of time, probably decades in many cases. There have been innumerable studies of the biological and molecular features of DCIS, especially since the 1970s. The cells of DCIS and invasive breast cancer are highly similar at the cellular and molecular levels, even though only one is invasive. Even at the genetic level, there are similarities: We are able to subdivide both invasive breast cancer and its non-invasive counterpart DCIS by molecular characteristics (based on features such as estrogen and progesterone receptor status (ER,PR), HER2, and grade).

Does all DCIS eventually progress to become invasive? We believe that not all DCIS will become invasive, but don't really know what percentage will do so. There are some small experiences of DCIS that was not treated; for example, there are limited studies of patients with DCIS that were originally misdiagnosed as benign, so they were not completely excised surgically. These retrospective studies suggest that in the modern era, at least a third or more DCIS cases will eventually progress to invasive breast cancer if undetected.

Size and type

The pathology report should address the size of the DCIS, preferably as measured under a microscope. The DCIS can affect your management recommendations. There are different patterns of low-grade (less aggressive-appearing) and moderate-grade DCIS:

- Papillary (abnormal cells protrude inwardly from the duct wall)
- Cribriform (Swiss cheese-appearance within the ducts)
- Solid (abnormal cells fill the ducts)

There is also high-grade DCIS, sometimes described as "comedo" or comedonecrosis. Comedo means that there are areas of dead (necrotic debris) abnormal cells inside the milk duct of the breast. As the cells are dividing rapidly they can't get enough nourishment, and these starving cells die, leaving areas of necrosis. Less common variants include the "clinging" carcinoma, intraductal signet ring carcinoma, and cystic hypersecretory duct carcinomas.

Margins

During a surgical biopsy or breast conserving surgery, your surgeon removes the DCIS and a surrounding zone of normal-appearing tissue. We refer to this healthy-looking tissue as the surgical margin. If you have no DCIS cells in the margin, it is likely that all of the DCIS has been removed, and we call the margins "negative" or uninvolved. If the margin is not clear, you may need to do more surgery to ensure that all of the measurable DCIS is removed.

Grade

The DCIS grade is a reflection of how fast the abnormal cells are growing. We typically grade DCIS as 1, 2 or 3. A low grade (grade 1) DCIS is growing slowly. A high grade DCIS is growing more rapidly. Many patients confuse grade and stage; grade is a measure of how aggressive the abnormal cells appear, while stage is a measure of the geographic extent of disease. Pure DCIS is Stage 0.

Size

The size of DCIS can be challenging to measure, as there is not typically a solid mass; rather, the DCIS often follows the branching structures along several milk ducts. The larger the DCIS, the higher the likelihood of having an associated microscopic component of invasive cancer.

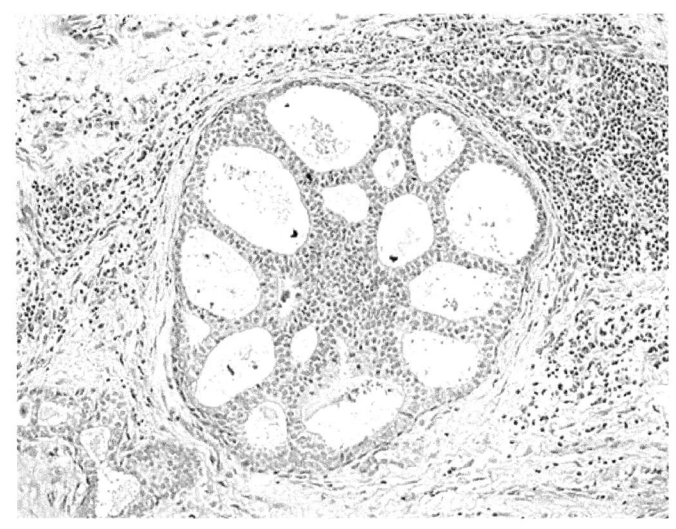

Cribriform DCIS

There are gaps between cancer cells in the affected breast ducts (like the pattern of holes in Swiss cheese).

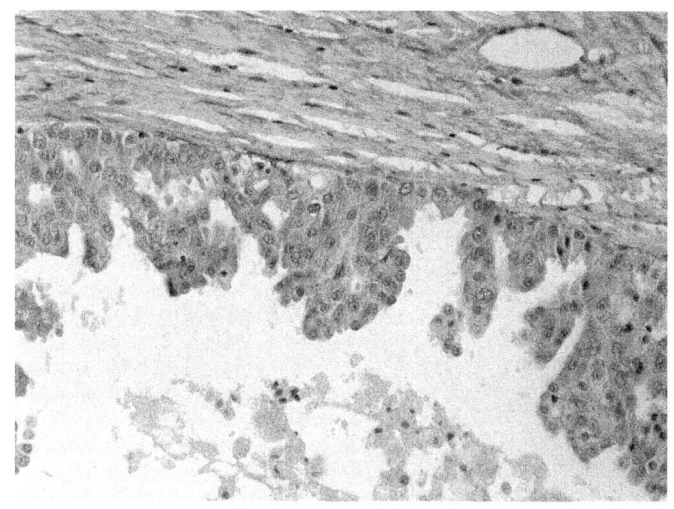

Papillary DCIS

The cancer cells are arranged in a finger-like pattern within the ducts. If the cells are very small, they are called micropapillary.

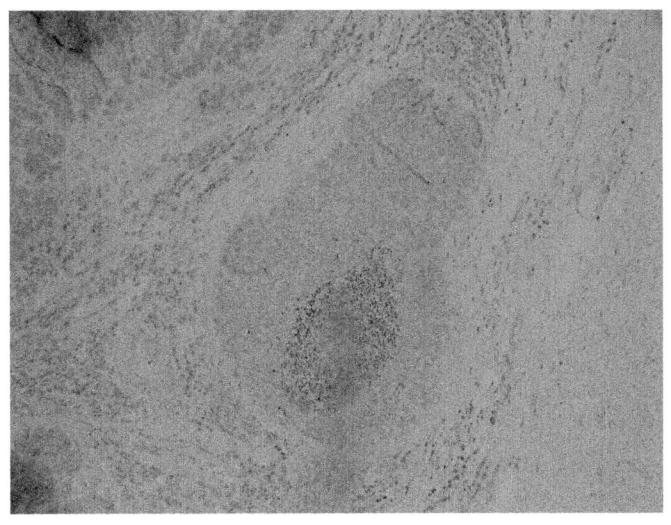

Comedo DCIS

High-grade DCIS is sometimes described as comedonecrosis. Comedo refers to areas of necrotic (dead) cancer cells, which build up inside the ducts. When cancer cells grow quickly, some cells don't get enough nourishment, with these starving cells then dying off, leaving areas of necrosis.

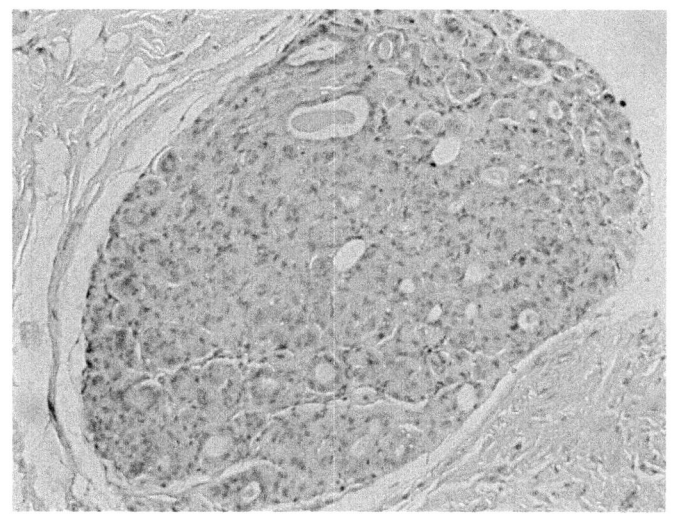

Solid DCIS

Cancer cells completely fill the affected breast ducts.

DCIS

Hormone (estrogen) receptors (ER)

The pathologist will test your DCIS for hormone receptor(s). These tests determine if your DCIS has receptors for the hormone estrogen. A positive result means that estrogen fuels the growth of the abnormal cells. If the DCIS is estrogen receptor positive (ER+), your doctor may recommend treatments to block the effects of estrogen or to lower your body's estrogen levels.

Classification

Many classification schemes have been proposed for DCIS. These often focus on the presence or absence of necrosis (cell breakdown) and characteristics of the cell nucleus (the nucleus stores the cell's DNA, and coordinates cell activities). On the previous pages, you saw reference to dividing DCIS into types based on the architectural pattern: Solid, cribriform, papillary, and micropapillary are examples. Today, **nuclear (central, DNA-containing parts of cells) grade** is emphasized, and is reported as low, intermediate, or high.

- Grade 1 (low-grade)
  Cells close to normal, and grow slowly.

- Grade 2 (intermediate grade)
  Cells appear abnormal, and grow faster than normal.

- Grade 3 (high grade)
  Cells appear very abnormal, and grow fast.

Estrogen receptors (ER) and progesterone receptors (PR) are uniformly expressed in normal breast tissue. Levels of ER tend to be higher in DCIS lesions that are less aggressive-appearing under the microscope. One review showed estrogen receptor expression in 83% of well-differentiated DCIS, 74% of poorly differentiated DCIS, 91% of DCIS lesions with no necrosis, and in 37% of DCIS lesions with significant necrosis. HER2 is not routinely checked.

DCIS: Are you sure?

The distinction between *low-grade* DCIS and atypical lesions that are not yet DCIS is primarily based on the extent of disease. The lesions may have similar histologic characteristics under the microscope. Perhaps not surprisingly, pathologists may misdiagnose breast tissue. A recent American study involved 115 pathologists and 240 breast biopsy specimens. Their diagnoses were matched against those of three experts. Here are the results:

- Pathologists correctly diagnosed abnormal, pre-cancer cells about half the time, no better than a coin toss.
- Pathologists mistakenly found something suspicious in 13 percent of normal tissue.
- 13% of DCIS cases were misdiagnosed as less serious, while **3 percent were mistaken for invasive cancer.**

HER2

Some cancers have a gene mutation that leads to the excess creation of the HER2 protein. The presence of HER2 can promote cell growth. HER2 over expression is seen more frequently in DCIS (particularly high-grade DCIS):

	HER2 +
• DCIS	50-60%
• Invasive ductal carcinoma	25-30%

While **we do not routinely test DCIS for HER2,** some data suggest that HER2-overexpressing DCIS is more likely to be associated with invasive breast cancer (compared with HER2-negative DCIS). In a University of Pennsylvania study, researchers found 37% of DCIS that had overexpression of HER2 had early invasive breast cancer associated with it. The chances of finding an associated invasive cancer increased by a factor of 6.4 with HER2 overexpression.

Margins

The American Society for Radiation Oncology, the Society of Surgical Oncology, and the American Society of Clinical Oncology concluded in 2016 that for DCIS: **A 2 millimeter clean margin is adequate for women treated with lumpectomy and whole breast radiation therapy.** Clean margins wider than 2 millimeters don't further reduce the risk of recurrence.

DCIS

Molecular profiling

While associated with a very high cancer-specific survival chance, ductal carcinoma *in situ* actually represents a group of diseases, with various prognoses and needs for treatment. In the future, we should be better able to understand who needs treatment (and who does not). Molecular profiling examines the genes, and offers the promise of more tailored management for DCIS in the future. Here are some factors that may influence DCIS prognosis: 1) p16 expression; 2) cyclooxygenase-2; and 3) Ki-67 proliferation index

In addition, the OncoType DX analyzes the activity of a group of genes in the DCIS to provide an individualized prediction of the 10-year risk of a future event (the return of DCIS or invasive cancer). This test can help some women with DCIS treated by surgery, with or without anti-estrogen therapy such as tamoxifen. While Medicare has established coverage for OncoType DX for women with DCIS, coverage outside Medicare varies by insurance plan.

How it works

The OncoType DX test works by examining a sample of the DCIS that has already been removed during the original surgery. The test measures a group of cancer genes to determine their activity. The result of the test is reported as a number between 0 and 100, known as the DCIS Score results. A lower DCIS Score result means that their is a lower chance that a tumor will come back in the same breast.

While the vast majority of patients with DCIS do not have an OncoType DX Breast DCIS test, the score can help some women determine how aggressive to be with treatment (radiation therapy? no radiation therapy?) One potential limitation of the use of the test is the fact that the study that validated it used cancer-free zones (margins) around the DCIS of at least 3 millimeters. The DCIS itself had to be 2.5 centimeters (2 inches) or smaller.

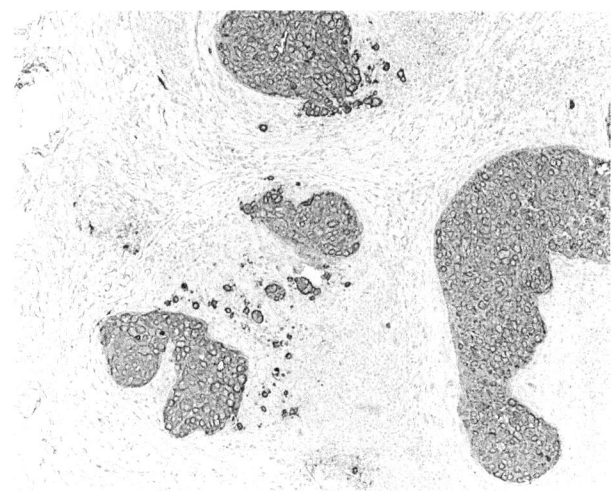

Microinvasion

Tumor (invasive component only) 1 mm or less in greatest dimension

Microinvasion is a term used to describe a borderline difference between the completely contained (with a duct) ductal carcinoma *in situ* (DCIS) and a minimally invasive ductal cancer. In essence, a very small amount of malignant cells are just beyond the duct lining, measuring less than one millimeter (1/25th of an inch). In cases with multiple foci of microinvasion (where no individual focus is larger than 1mm), the number of foci and range of sizes should be reported. We do not add the size of individual foci of microinvasion.

In the photomicrograph to the right, you can see abnormal cells that are stained to be brown in color. While most of the abnormal cells are confined to the ducts, there are small nests that have clearly escaped from the duct. Under the microscope, microinvasive breast carcinoma tends to be associated with high-grade DCIS and comedo-type necrosis. There is some evidence that the risk of microinvasion increases with larger size DCIS lesions and multicentric (in several areas of the breast) ones.

LCIS (lobular carcinoma in situ)

Lobular means that the abnormal cells start growing in the lobules, the milk-producing glands at the end of breast ducts. Carcinoma refers to any cancer that begins in the skin or other tissues that cover internal organs — such as breast tissue. *In situ* or "remaining in place" means that the abnormal growth remains inside the milk lobule and has not broken out into surrounding tissues. LCIS tends to affect more than one lobule.

Cancer?

Despite the fact that its name includes the term "carcinoma," LCIS is not a breast cancer. Rather, if you have LCIS, you are at higher risk for getting cancer in either breast at some point in the future. For this reason, some experts prefer the descriptor lobular neoplasia (a collection of abnormal cells) *in situ*. Fortunately, there are a variety of means to reduce your risk of the future development of cancer in either breast.

Uncommon

Lobular carcinoma *in situ* (LCIS) seems uncommon, but we don't know exactly how many people are affected. LCIS does not cause symptoms and usually does not show up on a mammogram. It tends to be found as a result of a breast biopsy performed for some other reason. LCIS is usually diagnosed before menopause, most commonly between the ages of 40 and 50. Less than 10 percent of women LCIS have already gone through menopause. LCIS is extremely uncommon among men.

Aggressive variant: Pleomorphic

There is evidence to support the existence of more aggressive variants of LCIS (for example, **pleomorphic LCIS**), which may have a greater potential than classic LCIS to develop into invasive lobular carcinoma. Some believe that pleomorphic marker not only increases the risk of a future cancer in either breast, but can sometimes evolve into an invasive cancer itself. You may consider complete excision with clear ("negative") margins for pleomorphic LCIS.

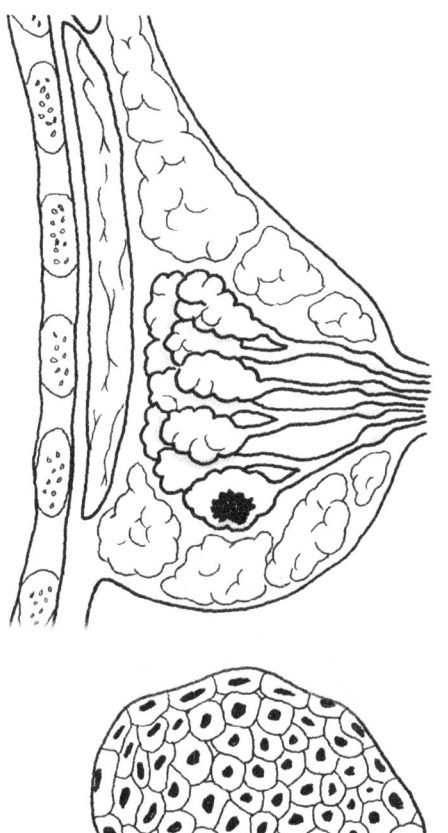

LCIS

LCIS

Necrosis

Necrosis means that some of the LCIS cells have died. Pleomorphic means that the LCIS cells look more atypical under the microscope than the usual case of LCIS. LCIS with either of these features (when compared to LCIS without them) may be more aggressive (grow faster and be more likely to spread) and appears to be associated with an even higher risk of invasive cancer. LCIS with either of these features may be treated differently than most cases of LCIS.

DCIS versus LCIS

Adhesion protein molecules are expressed in cells of epithelial* lineage. These are calcium-dependent cell-to-cell adhesion proteins. One of these adhesion molecules is known as epithelial cadherin (E-cadherin). Loss of E-cadherin is considered to be a basic defect in invasive lobular carcinoma of the breast. Not surprisingly, it is not fully expressed in pre-invasive disease; **loss of E-cadherin can help distinguish LCIS (loss) from DCIS (no loss).**

Microcalcifications

Calcifications may be associated with LCIS. Microcalcifications are mineral deposits that can be found in both non-cancerous and cancerous lesions. They can sometimes be seen both on mammograms and under the microscope. Because certain types of calcifications are found in areas containing cancer, their presence on a mammogram may lead to a biopsy of the area. Then, when the biopsy is done, the pathologist looks at the tissue removed to be sure that it contains calcifications. Microcalcifications and calcifications matter when they are found in areas containing cancer. When they are found alone (without worrisome changes in the breast ducts or lobules), they are not important.

***Epithelial tissues** line the cavities and surfaces of structures throughout the body. Many glands are made up of epithelial cells.

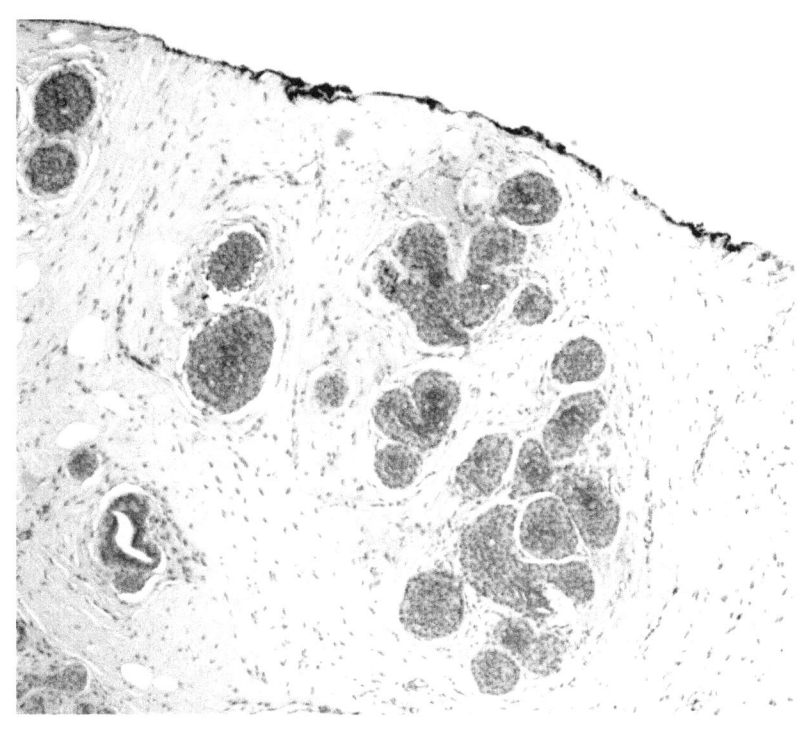

LCIS

Benign (not cancer)

Atypical hyperplasia (AH)

Hyperplasia describes an overgrowth (proliferation) of cells. It most often occurs inside the lobules or milk ducts. AH is a part of multistep process that can lead to breast cancer. First, the cells increase in number (hyperplasia), but still look normal. Then, they can progress to become atypical: The cells stack on top of one another, and begin to look abnormal. If the cells continue to change appearance and multiply, they can evolve into non-invasive *(in situ)* carcinoma. With in situ carcinoma, the cells remain confined to the area where they started growing (the ducts or lobules). Ultimately, progression to invasive cancer can occur.

Types

There are two main kinds of hyperplasia—usual and atypical. Both increase breast cancer risk, though atypical hyperplasia does so to a greater degree. For women with atypical hyperplasia (but not usual hyperplasia), there are special breast cancer screening and management recommendations.

Atypical hyperplasia is not a cancer, but rather a cell abnormality that increases your chance of breast cancer in the future. It can be the ductal type (atypical ductal hyperplasia; ADH) or the lobular type (atypical lobular hyperplasia; ALH). We do not know what causes atypical hyperplasia.

Increased risk

While atypical ductal hyperplasia (ADH) and atypical lobular hyperplasia (ALH) are *not* cancers, when present, they can markedly increase the risk of the development of a cancer in the breast in the future. In fact, atypical hyperplasia is associated with a 30% chance of getting breast cancer over the ensuing 25 years.

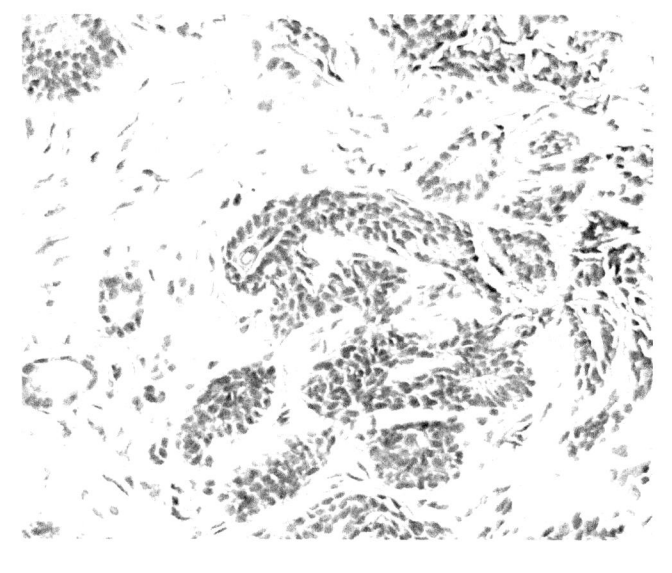

ADH

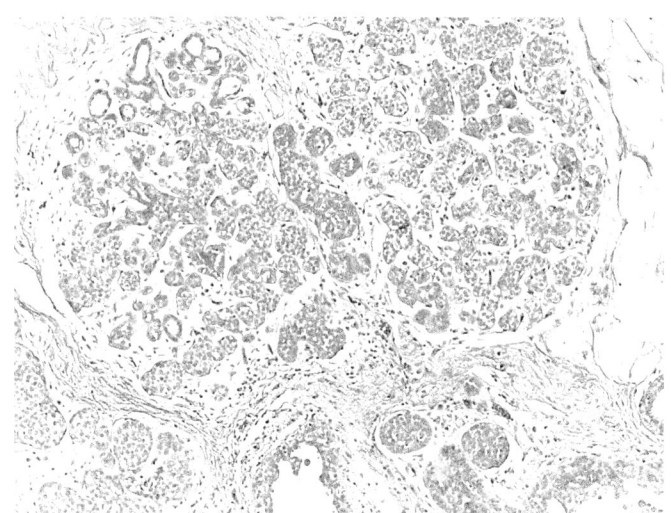

ALH

Benign (not cancer)

Simple cyst

This is the most common cause of a palpable mass. Cysts are benign (not cancer) fluid-filled sacs. They are more common among premenopausal women, and in their pure form do not increase the risk of breast cancer. Some cysts are palpable lumps in the breast, while others are not. If large enough, a cyst can cause pain. For women under 30 years-old, cysts are typically diagnosed with breast ultrasound (non-invasive imaging that uses sound waves). For non-pregnant women over 30, mammogram and/or a breast ultrasound may be used.

Management

Simple (uncomplicated) cysts often do not need treatment, as most disappear over time. Half are gone within a year, and 70 percent within five years. However, if the cyst causes pain or is large, it may be aspirated (drained) with a very thin needle. We do not yet have high level evidence to suggest that diet change can decrease your probability of developing cysts.

 If ultrasound testing suggests that the abnormality is *not* a simple fluid-filled cavity, you will likely need tissue removed (biopsy), or even to see a surgeon.

Lipoma

Lipomas are benign fatty tumors that can appear almost anywhere in the body, including the breast. They are typically non-tender, and may present as a somewhat squishy, non-tender lump. When in doubt, a biopsy can confirm the diagnosis.

Other benign lumps that are sometimes found in the breast include hamartomas, hemangiomas, hematomas, adenomyoepthelomas, and neurofibromas. None of these conditions raises breast cancer risk, but they may need to have a biopsy (tissue sampling) or removed to render a diagnosis.

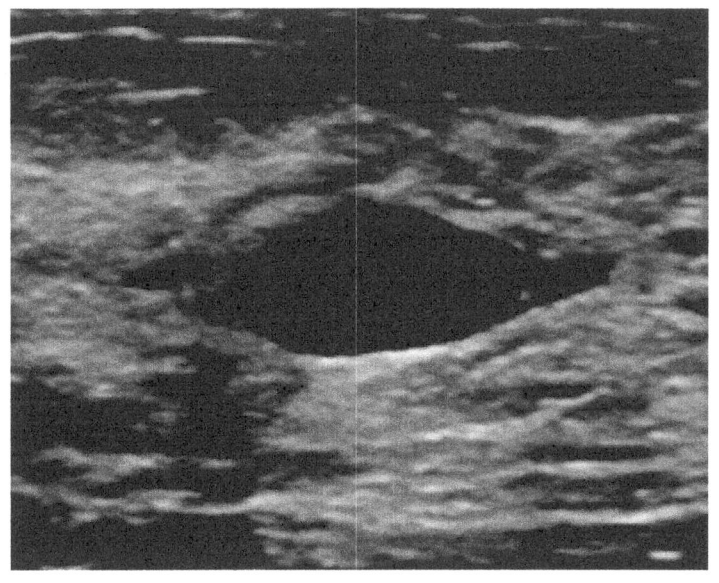

Cyst

Benign (not cancer)

Fibroadenoma

Fibroadenomas are solid masses that are **benign.** Women are often between ages 15 to 35. Most fibroadenomas do *not* increase your risk of developing breast cancer. However, there is a slight increase in risk for those with fibroadenoma who with a complex fibroadenoma, an associated proliferative disease, or a family history of breast cancer. Many recommend removal off fibroadenomas, especially if they are growing, cause discomfort, or change the breast shape. Sometimes, especially in middle-aged or elderly women, these tumors stop growing (or even shrink) without intervention. If your doctors feel certain the masses are fibroadenomas (and not breast cancer) and are not painful, fibroadenomas are often left in place and carefully monitored to make sure they don't grow.

Radial scar

Radial scars (also known as complex sclerosing lesions) have a core of connective tissue fibers. Milk ducts and lobules grow out from this core. Radial scars may appear similar to breast cancer on a mammogram, but radial scars are *not* cancer. Treatment consists of removal. Some (but not all) studies suggest that radial scars may increase your risk of a future breast cancer.

Adenosis (aggregate adenosis; adenosis tumor)

In adenosis the breast lobules are enlarged, and they contain more glands than usual. Adenosis is often found in biopsies of women with fibrocystic changes. There are many names for this condition, including aggregate adenosis, tumoral adenosis, or adenosis tumor. Even though some of these terms contain the term tumor, adenosis is *not* a cancer.

Sclerosing adenosis is a special type of adenosis in which the enlarged lobules are distorted by scar-like fibrous tissue. Some studies have associated sclerosing adenosis with a greater risk of developing breast cancer – about 1½ to 2 times the risk of women with no breast changes.

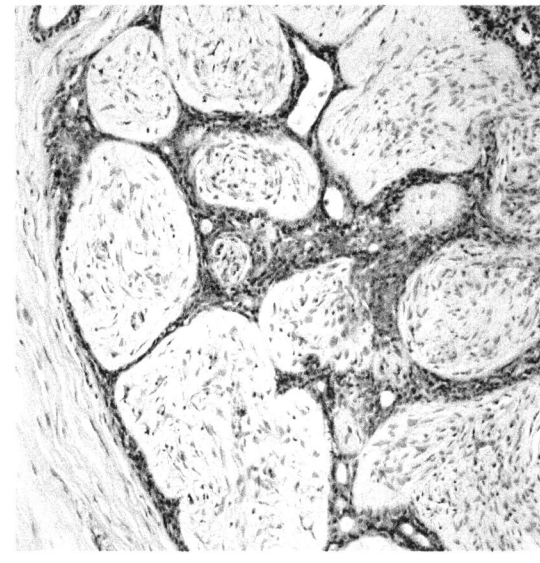

Fibroadenoma

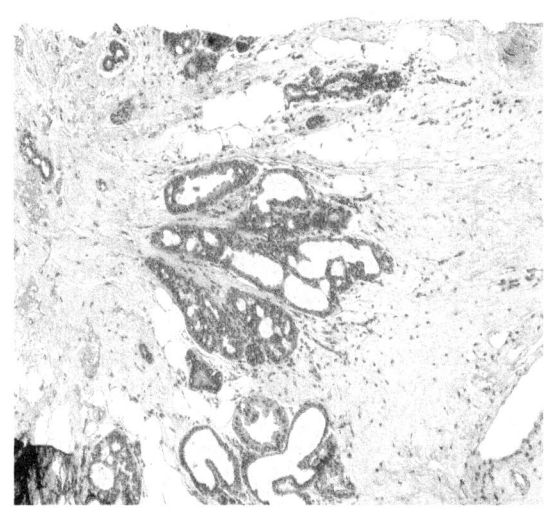

Radial scar

Benign (not cancer)

Phylloides

Phylloides tumors (full-OY-deez) are rare breast tumors that, like fibroadenomas, contain two types of breast tissue: stromal (connective) tissue and glandular (lobule and duct) tissue. They are most common in women in their 30s and 40s, but they may be found in women of any age.

Phylloides tumors are usually not true cancers, but in rare cases they may be. While up to one-third are classified as malignant based on how they look under the microscope, less than 5% of phylloides tumors overall are true cancers that spread to distant sites such as the lungs. Benign phylloides don't increase your future cancer risk. Malignant phylloides tumors are typically managed by removing them along with a wide margin of normal tissue (a margin), or by mastectomy (removing the entire breast) if needed. Close follow-up is required.

Intraductal papillomas

Intraductal papillomas are benign (not cancer) solid tumors that grow within the breast ducts. They are wart-like growths of gland tissue along with fibrous tissue and blood vessels. Solitary intraductal papillomas are a common cause of clear or bloody nipple discharge, especially when it comes from only one breast. Sometimes, they present as a small palpable lump behind or next to the nipple. They do not raise breast cancer risk unless there are other changes, such as atypical hyperplasia (AH).

Papillomas that are in small ducts in areas of the breast farther from the nipple may be multiple, and are less likely to cause nipple discharge. Papillomatosis is a type of hyperplasia in which there are very small areas of cell growth within the ducts, but they are not as distinct as papillomas. Finally, Papillomatosis is also linked to a slightly increased risk of breast cancer.

Atypical, palpable and multiple papillomas should be removed, as they will be upgraded to cancer up to 67 percent of the time.

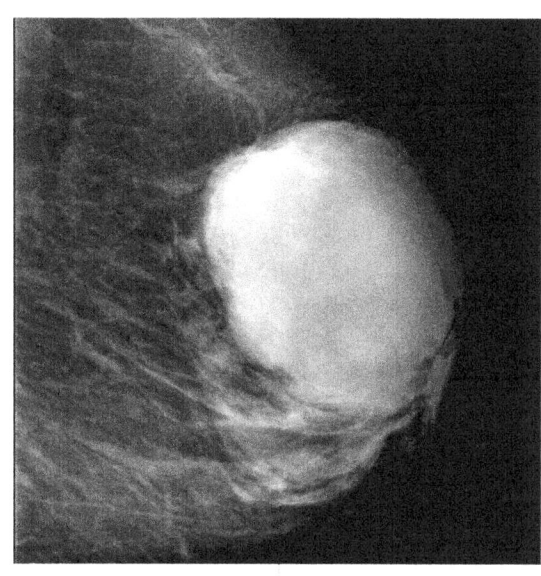

Phylloides
on mammogram

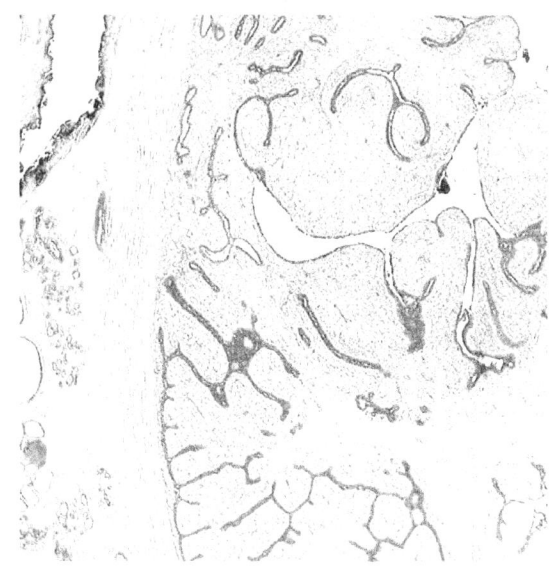

Phylloides
under the microscope

Fat necrosis and oil cysts

Here, typically as a result of injury to the breast, the tissue is damaged. Such injury may include radiation therapy directed at the breast, or surgery. Scar tissue can be the result. On occasion, scar tissue doesn't form in the usual way; instead, the fat cells die and release their contents. This forms a sac-like collection of greasy fluid called an oil cyst.

This oil cyst may be able to be felt (it is palpable), and can be challenging to discern from a true cancer by physical examination or mammograms. In this context, it is perhaps not surprising that a biopsy may be recommended.

Mastitis

Mastitis occurs when bacteria crawl through small openings of the eight to twelve breast ducts that are on the nipple surface. Mastitis begins as inflammation, but can evolve into a bacterial infection marked by redness, tenderness, and warmth of the breast. In more advanced situations, a lump (abscess) can form; essentially, this is a pocket of pus. We always **need to rule out inflammatory breast cancer** when we have mastitis that lasts more than a few days, in spite of appropriate treatment.

Mastitis is managed with warm compresses, acetaminophen and ibuprofen, breast massage, and antibiotics. Vibration therapy may also provide relief. Finally, a breast surgeon may be able to unclog ducts at the nipple surface and may use a thin needle to remove fluid (fine needle aspiration). Abscess management may include antibiotics and repeated aspirations or even drainage trough an open incision in the doctor's office or in the operating room.

 Mastitis does *not* raise your breast cancer risk. However, because an aggressive form of breast cancer (inflammatory breast cancer) can mimic mastitis, it is important to consider a biopsy if your symptoms do not improve within a week or so.

Hamartoma

These benign (not cancer) tumors are made up of the normal tissue found in the breast, but the cells grow in a disorganized fashion. These tumors can be soft and painless, but may grow to a large size. Often, because the cells are fairly normal appearing, a diagnosis may require a complete excision. While cancer is rarely associated with hamartoma, an excision confirms it.

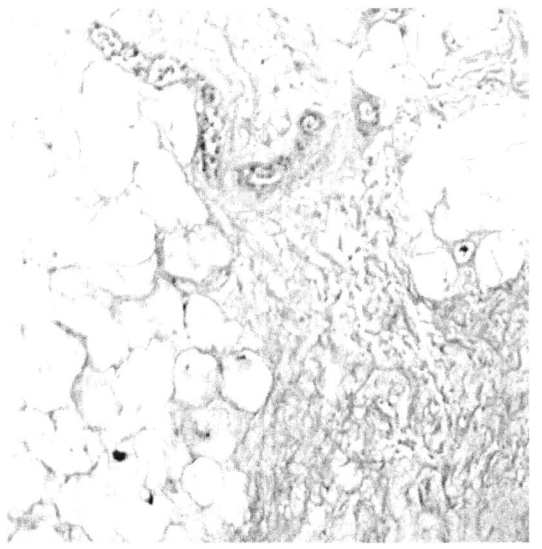

Fat necrosis

Benign (not cancer)

PASH

Pseudoangiomatous stromal hyperplasia (PASH) is sometimes mistaken for cancer. Under the microscope, PASH has small slits in the tissues that look like blood vessels, but aren't. Thuse the name pseudo (false) angiomatous (blood vessels). Alas, core needle biopsies with PASH may be mistaken for cancer; a second opinion from an expert pathologist should be considered. PASH is typically found incidentally with other biopsies, but sometimes presents as a palpable, non-tender thickening in the breast. PASH management is controversial. Excision may be indicated for enlarging masses or lesions with atypical features.

Duct ectasia

Mammary duct ectasia is common among women over 50. It occurs when a breast duct widens and its walls thicken, leading to a blockage and fluid build-up. It may be found when you are having a biopsy for a separate condition. Less commonly, you may experience a thick green or black discharge, with the nipple becoming tender, red, or pulled inward. A hard lump may develop because of the scar tissue that is forming.

This condition sometimes improves without treatment, or with warm compresses and antibiotics. If the symptoms do not go away, the abnormal duct may be removed with surgery. Ectasia itself does *not* raise your risk of cancer.

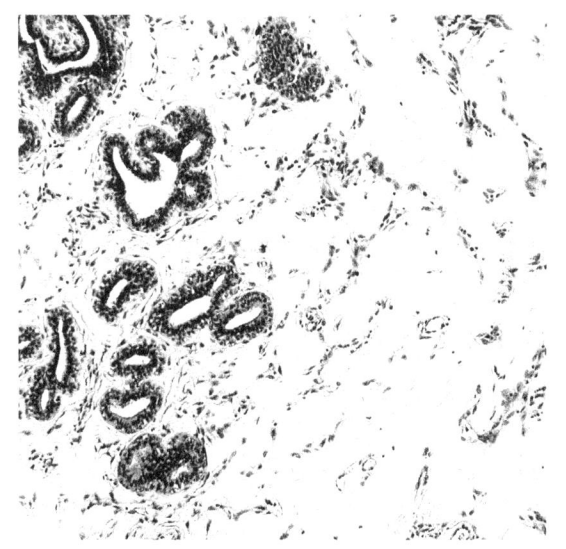

PASH
under the microscope

Paget's disease

Paget's disease of nipple

In 1874, Sir James Paget described 15 women with chronic nipple ulceration who all developed breast cancer within two years. While Paget believed the nipple changes were themselves benign (not cancer) we subsequently discovered that the characteristic cells in the outer layer of the cells covering the nipple were indeed malignant. Please note that Paget's disease of the nipple a different entity than is Paget'sdisease of the bone.

Presentation

An underlying breast cancer (in situ or invasive) is present in up to nearly 90 percent of the time, although there may or may not be an associated breast mass or mammogram abnormality. A palpable breast mass is associated with Paget's in about 50 percent of cases, with the mass often more than 2 cm from the nipple/areaola. In 20 percent of cases, there is a mammogram abnormality, but no palpable mass. A quarter witll have no underlying mass or mammogram abnormality, but there is an occult breast cancer. Finally about 12 to 15 percent of cases are not associated with a palpable mass, mammogram abnormality, or cancer in the main breast tissue.

Skin biopsy

A nipple scraping can accurately diagnosis Paget's, but the diagnosis is more commonly made after a punch biopsy or wedging of the nipple. The hallmark of Paget's disease of the nipple is the presence of cancer cells (Paget cells) occuring singly or in small groups within the nipple outer layer of cells. Sometimes, the cells can have a similar appearance to melanoma. In cases where we are not sure what type of cancer is seen, more advanced testing (such as so-called immunochemistry) may be done.

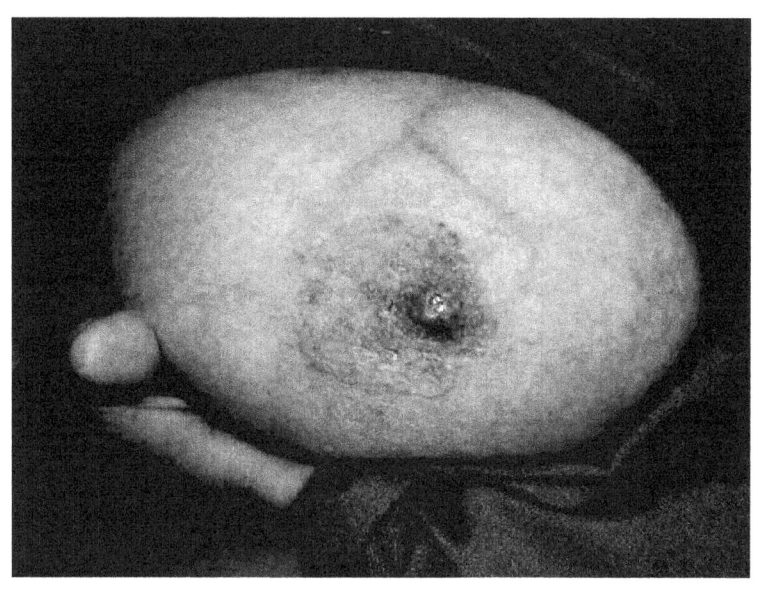

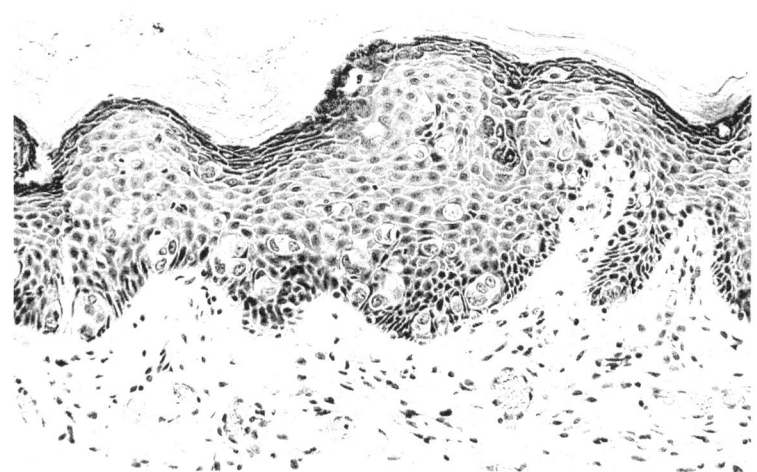

Paget's disease of the nipple
Paget cells are large cells with a clear halo

Margins

noun mar·gin \\'mär-jin\\
a rim of normal breast tissue surrounding a suspicious area

At surgery, a rim of normal breast tissue (a margin) surrounding the suspicious area is taken out to be sure the entire measurable tumor is removed. When a tumor is removed, some tissue surrounding it is also removed. The tumor with surrounding tissue is rolled in a special ink so that the outer edges, or margins, are clearly visible under a microscope. A pathologist reports the margins:

- **Positive margins** (ink on invasive carcinoma or ductal carcinoma *in situ*) are associated with a two-fold increase in the risk of in-breast relapse compared to negative (clear) margins. This increased risk is not mitigated by favorable biology, endocrine therapy or a radiation boost.

- **More widely clear margins** than no ink on tumor do not significantly decrease the rate of in-breast recurrence. There is no evidence that more widely clear margins reduce recurrence for young patients, unfavorable biology, lobular cancers, or cancers with an extensive intraductal component. Finally, classic LCIS at the margin is not an indication for re-excision. The significance of pleomorphic LCIS at the margin remains uncertain.

The optimal cancer-free zone for a lumpectomy is controversial. In this context, an expert consensus panel considered a meta-analysis of 33 studies (with 28,162 patients) examining margin width and in-breast recurrence. Researchers also looked at results of randomized clinical trials, reproducibility of margin assessment, and current patterns of multimodality care. They concluded that **clear margins, no matter how small as long as there is no ink on the cancer tumor, should be the standard for lumpectomy** surgery. These guidelines apply to *invasive* cancer, Stages I and II managed with breast-conserving surgery followed by whole breast radiation therapy.

Margin width?

The American Society for Radiation Oncology and the Society of Surgical Oncology concluded in 2016 that

Use of a **2 millimeter margin as the standard** for an adequate margin in DCIS treated with whole-breast irradiation is associated with lower rates of in-breast recurrence and has the potential to decrease re-excision rates, improve cosmetic outcomes, and decrease health care costs. Clinical judgment should be used in determining the need for further surgery in patients with negative margins narrower than 2 millimeters.

Estrogen receptors

ER / PR

Your biopsy or surgical material will be tested to see if your breast cancer cells have receptors for the hormones estrogen and progesterone. Hormone receptors are proteins — found in and on breast cells — that pick up hormone signals telling the cells to grow.

A cancer is estrogen receptor-positive (or ER+) if it has receptors for estrogen. This suggests that the cancer cells, like normal breast cells, receive signals from estrogen that promote their growth. The cancer is progesterone receptor-positive (PR+) if it has progesterone receptors; that is, the cancer cells receive signals from progesterone that promote their growth. DCIS may or not be tested for PR. Just over two-thirds of breast cancers test positive for hormone receptors.

Why is ER status important?

Hormone receptor status indicates whether your cancer is likely to respond to endocrine (anti-hormonal) therapy. Endocrine therapy approaches include medications that either (1) lower the amount of estrogen in your body or (2) block estrogen from supporting the growth and function of breast cells. If the breast cancer cells have hormone receptors, then these medications can slow stop their growth. If the cancer is hormone-receptor-negative (no receptors are present), then hormonal therapy would not work. You and your doctor can then select other types of treatment.

Estrogen receptors (ER): Understanding your results

A test should be done for estrogen receptors. If your result is reported as "positive" or "negative," ask your doctor for a specific number. Different labs have varying cutoff points for calling a cancer hormone receptor-positive versus hormone receptor-negative. Even cancers with low numbers of hormone receptors may respond to anti-hormonal therapy targeting estrogen.

ESTROGEN hormone fuels the growth and division of some breast cancer cells

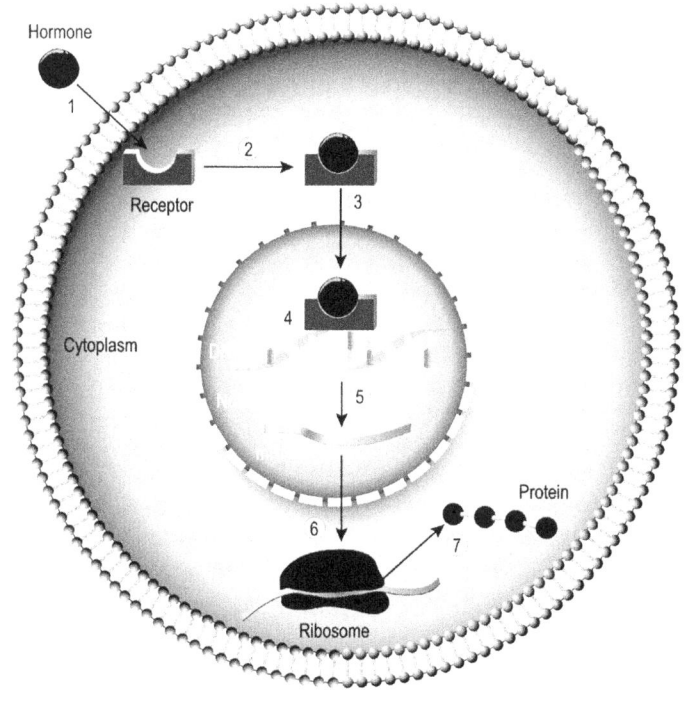

Ask

- **Where**

    Where is my cancer located in the breast?

- **What**

    Can you explain my pathology report to me? What cancer type do I have? Is my breast cancer estrogen receptor positive (ER +)? What is my DCIS grade? What does that mean for me?

- **Copies**

    Can I have a copy of my pathology report?

- **Second opinions**

    Most insurance plans will allow you to get an additional opinion, especially if the second health care provider is a member of your health plan. I think it may be especially important to get a second opinion for for the low-grade type of ductal carcinoma *in situ* (DCIS). Sometimes that opinion is best obtained from an expert in pathology, reviewing the slides containing the material from your surgery.

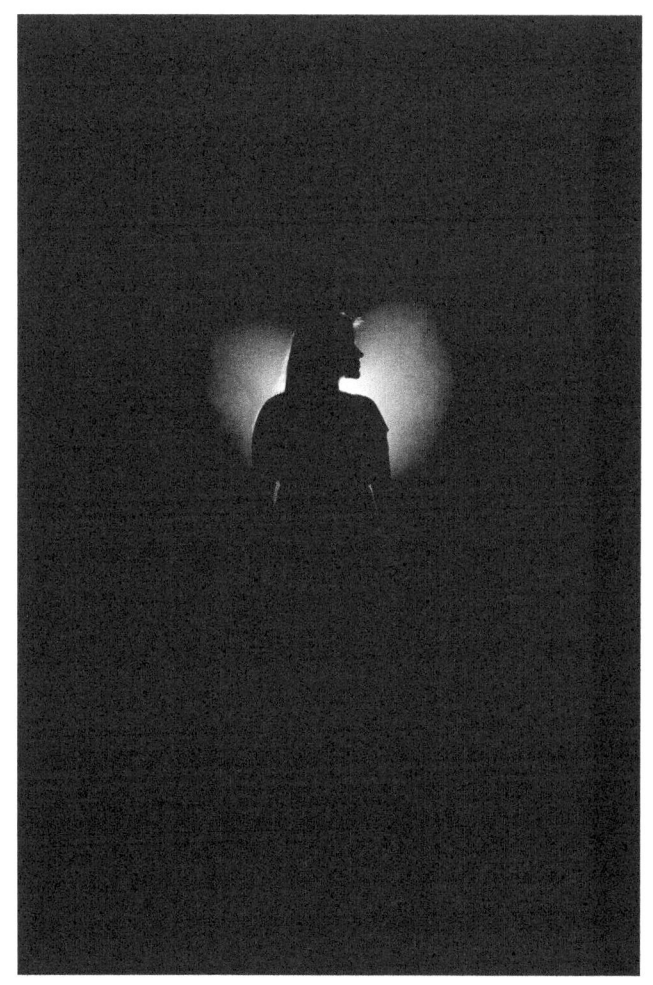

STAGE
CANCER EXTENT

Stage

The stage describes the **extent of cancer** in the body. Your stage is based on whether the cancer is invasive or non-invasive, the tumor size, the number of lymph nodes involved (if any), and whether the cancer has spread to distant parts of the body. Stage is one of the most important factors in determining prognosis and management options. Staging provides a common language for health care team members to effectively communicate about a patient's cancer and to collaborate on the best courses of management. Understanding the cancer's stage is also critical to identifying clinical trials that may be appropriate for particular patients.

Testing

Depending on the results of your physical exam and biopsy, your doctor may want you to have certain imaging tests such as a chest x-ray, mammograms of both breasts, bone scans, computed tomography (CT) scans, magnetic resonance imaging (MRI), and/or positron emission tomography (PET) scans. Blood tests may also be done to evaluate your overall health and can uncommonly indicate if the cancer has spread to certain organs.

TNM (T is for Tumor, N is for Nodes, M is for Metastases)

We use a staging system that allows us to summarize the extent of cancer in a clear way. The most common system used to describe the stages of breast cancer is the American Joint Committee on Cancer (AJCC) TNM system.

- **Clinical Stage**
  Your clinical stage is based on your physical exam, biopsy, and imaging.

- **Pathologic stage**
  Your pathologic stage uses information from the clinical stage, but adds in the findings from surgery (for example, how many lymph nodes are involved with cancer, if any nodes were removed).

Staging

Metastases

Symptoms can include significant weight loss, unusual bone pain, a chronic cough, and shortness of breath can be symptoms of metastases.

Testing

All patients should have their DCIS tested for **estrogen receptors, as well as mammograms of both breasts.** Selected patients may have genetic counseling (if the patient is at risk for hereditary breast cancer) and/or MRI of both breasts.

The stages of breast cancer range from 0 to IV (0 to 4). We determine the overall stage by looking at three factors:

- **T** (Tumor size)
- **N** (Lymph node status)
- **M** (Metastases)

- Clinical staging is determined before surgery
- Pathologic staging is determined after surgery

T is for Tumor

TX: Stage cannot be assessed	
T0: No tumor found	
Tis: Carcinoma *in situ* (*in situ* means remaining in place)	**Tis (DCIS):** Ductal carcinoma *in situ* **Tis (Paget):** Paget disease of the nipple
T1: Tumor 2 cm or less	**T1mi:** 0.1 cm or smaller **T1a:** Over 0.1 cm, but no larger than 0.5 cm **T1b:** Larger than 0.5 cm, but no larger than 1 cm **T1c:** Larger than 1 cm, but no larger than 2 cm
T2: Tumor over 2 cm, but no larger than 5 cm	
T3: Tumor over 5 cm	
T4: Tumor any size, but has spread beyond the breast to the chest wall and/or skin	**T4a:** Tumor spread to the chest wall **T4b:** Tumor spread to the skin, but is not inflammatory breast cancer **T4c:** Tumor spread to the chest wall *and* skin **T4d:** Inflammatory breast cancer

N is for Nodes
Clinical (before surgery)

NX: Regional nodes cannot be assessed (e.g., they were previously removed)

N0: No regional node metastases

N1: Metastases to movable ipsilateral level I, II axillary node(s)

N2a: Spread to ipsilateral level I, II axillary nodes fixed to one another (matted)
or to other structures

N2b: Spread to ipsilateral internal mammary nodes
and in the absence of clinically evident level I, II axillary node metastases

N3a Spread to ipsilateral infraclavicular lymph node(s)
N3b Spread to ipsilateral internal mammary lymph node(s) and axillary node(s)
N3c Metastases in ipsilateral supraclavicular (above collar bone) node(s)

N is for Nodes
Pathologic (after surgery)

pNX Regional nodes cannot be assessed

pN0 Cancer has not spread to nearby nodes*

pN1mi: Micrometastases (tiny areas of cancer spread) in 1 to 3 lymph nodes under the arm. The areas of cancer spread in the lymph nodes are 2 mm or less across (but at least 200 cancer cells or 0.2mm across).

pN1a: Cancer spread to 1 to 3 nodes under the arm with at least one area of cancer spread greater than 2 mm across.

pN1b: Cancer spread to internal mammary nodes, but spread only in sentinel node biopsy (it did not cause the nodes to become enlarged).

pN1c: Both N1a and N1b apply.

pN2a: Cancer spread to 4 to 9 lymph nodes under the arm, with at least one area of cancer spread larger than 2 mm.

pN2b: Cancer spread to one or more internal mammary lymph nodes, causing them to become enlarged.

pN3a: Cancer spread to 10 or more axillary lymph nodes, with at least one area of cancer spread greater than 2 mm, or cancer has spread to the lymph nodes under the collarbone, with at least one area of cancer spread over 2 mm.

pN3b: Cancer in at least one axillary node (with at least one area of cancer spread greater than 2 mm) and in internal mammary lymph nodes, or cancer spread to 4 or more axillary lymph nodes (with at least one area of cancer spread greater than 2 mm), and tiny amounts of cancer are found in internal mammary nodes on sentinel lymph node biopsy.

pN3c: Cancer has spread to the nodes above the collarbone with at least one area of cancer spread greater than 2 mm.

M is for Metastasis

M0: No distant spread is found on x-rays (or other imaging procedures) or by physical exam.*

M1: Cancer has spread to distant organs. The most common sites are bone, lung, and liver, and brain.

* cM0 (i+): Small numbers of cancer cells are found in blood or bone marrow (using special, non-routine tests), or tiny areas of cancer spread (no larger than 0.2mm) are found in lymph nodes away from the underarm, collarbone, or internal mammary areas.

About 5 percentage of U.S. women will have metastatic disease when they are first diagnosed with breast cancer. The majority of those with metastases have been previously treated, and the breast cancer has returned and spread to distant sites.

Putting it all together

Stage 0 (DCIS)	Tis	N0	M0

Early breast cancer			
Stage IA	T1	N0	M0
Stage IB	T0-1	N1mi	M0
	T1	N1mi	M0
Stage IIA	T0	N1	M0
	T1	N1	M0
	T2	N0	M0
Stage IIB	T2	N1	M0
	T3	N0	M0

Locally advanced breast cancer			
Stage IIIA	T0	N2	M0
	T1	N2	M0
	T2	N2	M0
	T3	N1	M0
	T3	N2	M0
Stage IIIB	T4	N0	M0
	T4	N1	M0
	T4	N2	M0
Stage IIIC	Any T	N3	M0

Metastatic breast cancer			
Stage IV	Any T	Any N	M1

Metastases

For those with DCIS, tests are *not* done to check for cancer spread to distant organs such as the bones, lungs or liver.

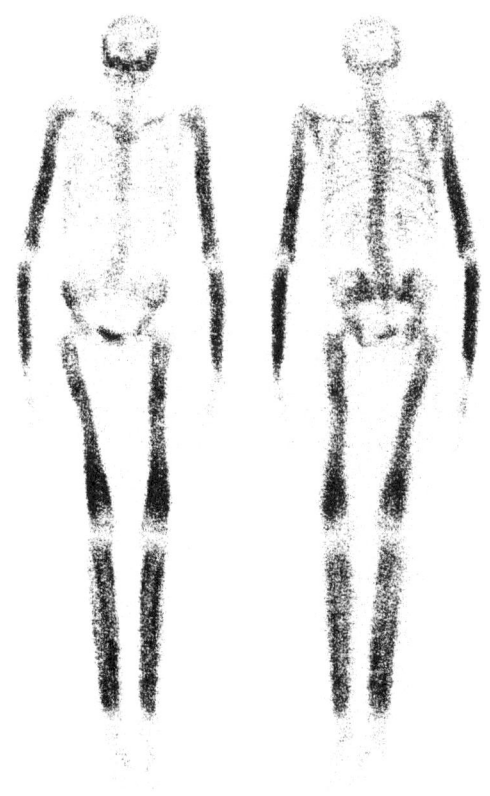

Metastasis
Cancer spread to distant organs, such as the bones, lungs or liver.

Staging

New and improved system

In 2017, the American Joint Committee on Cancer (AJCC) updated the staging system for breast cancer. **Stage** refers to the amount of cancer (size of the main tumor, spread to lymph nodes or to distant sites). Now, the definitions of each stage vary depending on cancer type. Cancer stage often correlates with outcomes, and management recommendations usually take into account the stage of disease.

Incorporating cancer cell biology

As our knowledge of tumor biology increases, it has become clear that stage is not the only factor that impacts prognosis. Tumor biology and behavior are very important, and in some cases may be more important than stage. A small tumor with aggressive behavior characteristics may may result in worse outcomes compared to a larger, but slower growing cancer.

Prognostic stage group

The 8th version of the AJCC staging system for breast cancer now takes into account tumor biology. Factors such as cell grade, estrogen receptor and HER2 status, grade, and (if performed) tumor genomic tests such as OncoType DX are now incorporated into the clinical (before surgery) and pathological (after surgery) prognostic stage. Taking into account these biologic factors means that the stage will have more meaningful prognostic information. Some larger tumors will now be considered stage I, and some smaller lesions will be upstaged based on their biology. In a large validation study performed by researchers at the University of Texas MD Anderson Cancer Center, 31% of patients were upstaged, and 20% of patients were downstaged. The updated prognostic stage performed better (in terms of predicting patient outcomes) than the standard anatomic stage. The pathologic prognostic stage is not applicable to patients receiving neoadjuvant therapy. Many patients with triple negative and HER2-positive beast cancer receive neoadjuvant chemotherapy.

Pathologic Prognostic Stage

TNM	Grade	HER2	ER	PR	Prognostic Stage Group
Tis N0 M0	Any	Any	Any	Any	**0**
T1* N0 M0 T0 N1mi M0 T1* N1mi M0	G1	Any	Any	Any	**IA**
	G2 or G3	Positive	Any	Any	**IA**
		Negative	Positive	Any	**IB**
		Negative	Negative		**IB**
T0 N1** M0 T1* N1** M0 T2 N0 M0	G1	Positive	Positive	Positive	**IA**
				Negative	**IB**
			Negative	Positive	**IB**
				Negative	**IIA**
		Negative	Positive	Positive	**IA**
				Negative	**IB**
			Negative	Positive	**IB**
				Negative	**IIA**
	G2	Positive	Positive	Positive	**IA**
				Negative	**IB**
			Negative	Positive	**IB**
				Negative	**IIA**
		Negative	Positive	Positive	**IA**
				Negative	**IIA**
			Negative	Any	**IIA**
	G3	Positive	Positive	Positive	**IA**
				Negative	**IIA**
			Negative	Any	**IIA**
		Negative	Positive	Positive	**IB**
				Negative	**IIA**
			Negative	Any	**IIA**

Pathologic Prognostic Stage

TNM	Grade	HER2	ER	PR	Prognostic Stage Group
T2 N1*** M0 T3 N0 M0	G1	Positive	Positive	Positive	IA
				Negative	IIB
			Negative	Any	IIB
		Negative	Positive	Positive	IA
				Negative	IIB
			Negative	Any	IIB
	G2	Positive	Positive	Positive	IB
				Negative	IIB
			Negative	Any	IIB
	G3	Positive	Positive	Positive	IB
				Negative	IIB
			Negative	Any	IIB
		Negative	Positive	Positive	IIA
				Negative	IIB
			Negative	Positive	IIB
				Negative	IIIA
T0 N2 M0 T1* N2 M0 T2 N2 M0 T3 N1*** M0 T3 N2 M0	G1	Positive	Positive	Positive	IB
				Negative	IIIA
			Negative	Any	IIIA
		Negative	Positive	Positive	IB
				Negative	IIIA
			Negative	Any	IIIA
	G2	Positive	Positive	Positive	IB
				Negative	IIIA
			Negative	Any	IIIA

Pathologic Prognostic Stage

TNM	Grade	HER2	ER	PR	Stage Group
T0 N2 M0 T1 N2 M0 T1mic N2 M0 T2 N2 M0 T3 N1* M0 T3 N2 M0	G3	Positive	Positive	Positive	**IIA**
				Negative	**IIIA**
			Negative	Any	**IIIA**
		Negative	Positive	Positive	**IIB**
				Negative	**IIIA**
			Negative	Positive	**IIIA**
				Negative	**IIIC**
T4 N0 M0 T4 N1** M0 T4 N2 M0 Any T N3 M0	G1	Positive	Positive	Positive	**IIIA**
				Negative	**IIIB**
			Negative	Any	**IIIB**
		Negative	Positive	Positive	**IIIA**
				Negative	**IIIB**
			Negative	Any	**IIIB**
	G2	Positive	Positive	Positive	**IIIA**
				Negative	**IIIB**
			Negative	Any	**IIIB**
		Negative	Positive	Positive	**IIIA**
				Negative	**IIIB**
			Negative	Negative	**IIIC**
			Negaitve	Positive	**IIIB**
	G3	Positive	Any	Any	**IIIB**
		Negative			
Any T Any N M1	Any	Any	Any	Any	**IV**

* N1 does not include N1mi. T1, N1mi, M0 and T0, N1mi, M0 are included for prognostic staging with T1, N0, M0 cancers of the same prognostic factor status.

** N1 includes N1mi. T2, T3, and T4 cancers and N1mi are included for prognostic staging with T2, N1; T3, N1; and T4, N1, respectively.

Note: If performed, when OncoType DX score is less than 11 for T1-2, N0, M0 disease, if HER 2 negative, the Pathologic Prognostic Group is IA.

PROGNOSIS

DCIS

Survival

Researchers used the Surveillance, Epidemiology and End Results (SEER) database to study women diagnosed with DCIS from 1988 to 2011. The study included 108,196 women whose risk of dying of breast cancer was compared with that of women in the general population. The average age at diagnosis for women was nearly 54 and the average duration of follow-up was 7.5 years.

10-year survival is 99%
The 10-year disease-specific survival probability following treatment for DCIS was 98.9%. By the 20 year mark, it dropped to 96.7%. The long-term death rate appeared to be higher for women who received a diagnosis before age 35 compared with older women (7.8 percent vs. 3.2 percent) and for black women compared with non-Hispanic white women (7 percent vs. 3 percent).

The authors note the finding of "greatest clinical importance" was that preventing an ipsilateral (on the same side of the body) invasive recurrence did *not* prevent death from breast cancer. Among all patients, the risk of ipsilateral invasive recurrence at 20 years was 5.9 percent and the risk of contralateral invasive recurrence was 6.2 percent.

Higher risk features
Your pathology report after a breast biopsy and after surgery tell you and your doctor the features of your DCIS. Even if you have several high-risk features, you may never develop invasive breast cancer. Higher risk features include:

- DCIS is in more than one area of your breast
- DCIS is high grade
- DCIS margins are suboptimal (for example, involved)
- Young age at diagnosis: The US SEER database showed a **3.2% risk breast cancer-related death for a patient found with DCIS at 35 years old or later; for those under 35, the risk was 7.8 percent.**

99%

That's the 10-year odds of surviving DCIS. The **20-year breast cancer-specific survival is 96.7 percent.**

DCIS

Local (in-breast) control

Local control

- Lumpectomy +/- radiation therapy

For women who had a lumpectomy, radiation therapy reduces the risk of developing an ipsilateral invasive recurrence (2.5 percent vs. 4.9 percent) but does *not* reduce breast cancer-specific death chances at 10 years (0.8 percent vs. 0.9 percent).

- Mastectomy

Patients who have a unilateral (single breast) mastectomy have a lower risk of an in-breast invasive recurrence at 10 years, compared to patients who have a lumpectomy (1.3 percent vs. 3.3 percent) but have a higher breast cancer-specific death rate (1.3 percent vs. 0.8 percent).

These data are from the US Surveillance, Epidemiology and End Results (SEER) database. The bottom line? Adding radiation therapy to lumpectomy reduces the local recurrence risk by half, but does *not* improve survival odds. A mastectomy yields a very low local recurrence rate at about 1%, but has survival chances similar to a breast-preserving approach to management.

- Adding estrogen "blockers" to lumpectomy

The use of drugs such as tamoxifen after lumpectomy and radiation therapy can reduce the risk of cancer in the opposite breast by about half, and can lower the same breast risk by about a third.

On the next page, we will turn to some of the individual studies (as well as meta-analysis, or collection of studies) to get a better sense of the roles of radiation therapy and/or endocrine therapy after breast-conserving surgery.

Radiation therapy (after lumpectomy)

High level evidence for RT (in-breast control benefit)

A meta-analysis (an analysis of a collection of studies) of four large multicenter randomized trials confirmed the results of the individual trials: **Adding radiation therapy to breast-conserving surgery for DCIS significantly cuts the chances of a subsequent event in the same breast.** Rates of local failure at median follow-up intervals of approximately 13 to 17 years were 25% to 35% in the unirradiated arms compared with 10% to 20% in the irradiated arms. The National Surgical Adjuvant Breast and Bowel Project (NSABP) B-17 trial is illustrative:

- At a median follow-up of 17.25 years, compared with lumpectomy alone, radiation therapy lowered the chances of a future invasive cancer in the same breast (crude local recurrence 20% versus 35%).
- Adding radiation therapy did *not* improve survival odds.

Are these studies relevant today? A contrarian view

Dr. Abram Recht of Harvard has an interesting take on whether the four first-generation randomized trials in DCIS are still relevant. So many aspects of patient evaluation and selection for breast-conserving therapy were different then than they are now; for example, there was much less use of magnification mammography, with resultant potential underestimation of the extent of DCIS. Pathologic evaluation was not standardized, and only limited sampling was performed even with large specimens. Here is Dr. Recht's reply to the question of whether the studies noted above are valuable today:

> Yes—they showed that RT substantially reduced local failure rates, (but did not change the risk of metastases or breast cancer death). And no—even though life-threatening adverse effects of RT are rare, its ability to reduce the absolute risk of local recurrence is much smaller [than historically] for many (perhaps most) patients presenting today with ductal carcinoma *in situ*.

DCIS

Local (in-breast) control

Margins

A surgical margin is a cancer-free zone around the removed DCIS. Uninvolved margins lower the risk that the DCIS will return in the same place. Let's look at some of the available data.

- Meta-analysis (analysis of a collection of studies)

In a meta-analysis of 4660 patients with DCIS treated with breastconserving surgery and radiation, a surgical margin of less than 2 millimeters (mm) was associated with increased rates of local recurrence compared with margins of 2mm or more. There were no differences when comparing margins greater than 5mm to margins of 2mm.

- Retrospective study

A large, retrospective study found that close margins (2mm or less) did *not* increase local recurrence rates, compared to a margin of 2mm.

So, what is the optimal margin for DCIS to reduce local recurrence after breast-conserving surgery? There is not yet a clear answer, but I generally prefer to see 2mm (or more) margins, *when possible.* At surgery, you should have a specimen radiograph (X-ray picture of the tissue removed), as it can confirm that all mammographically-detectable DCIS has been excised.

The National Comprehensive Cancer Network (NCCN) Panel agrees that patients should have a complete resection documented by an analysis of margins and with specimen radiographs (X-rays taken, during the surgery, of the removed tissue). If there is any uncertainty about the adequacy of the excision margins, the patient should have a repeat mammogram after surgery. Finally, clips are typically placed by the surgeon to demarcate the biopsy area.

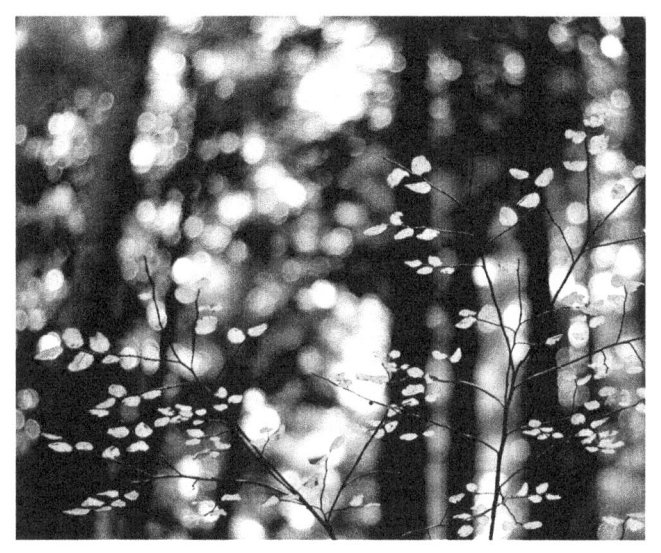

DCIS

Endocrine (anti-estrogen) therapy

Adding tamoxifen pills
Tamoxifen drops the risk of cancer events in both breasts (but does not improve survival odds). Let's look at the results of an important clinical trial that randomized women with DCIS (who had lumpectomy and radiation therapy) to the anti-estrogen pill tamoxifen for 5 years versus a placebo (a pill with no activity). Here are the results after a median follow-up of 13.6 years:

- Same breast risk reduction: Tamoxifen led to a 3.4% absolute reduction in ipsilateral (same) breast events.*

- Opposite breast risk reduction: Tamoxifen led to a 3.2% absolute reduction in contralateral (opposite) breast events.**

- Tamoxifen did *not* improve survival odds.

Other anti-estrogen pills
Researchers found that anastrazole (Arimidex) was better than tamoxifen at reducing recurrence risk among post-menopausal women diagnosed with hormone-receptor-positive DCIS.

---

* **Tamoxifen** led to a 10-year cumulative rate of 4.6% for invasive and 5.6% for non-invasive breast cancers in the ipsilateral (same) breast compared with 7.3% for invasive and 7.2% for non-invasive breast cancers in placebo-treated women.

**The cumulative 10-year frequency of invasive and non-invasive breast cancer in the contralateral (opposite) breast was 6.9% and 4.7% in the placebo and tamoxifen groups, respectively. No differences in overall survival (OS) were noted.

Tamoxifen versus anastrozole for DCIS

Here are the 10-year results for events in the same or opposite breast (Remember that we can only use anastrazole if you have already gone through menopause) for individuals who have DCIS:

- Anastrozole (Arimidex)
93.5% of the women had **no** recurrence

- Tamoxifen
89.2% of the women had **no** recurrence

Under 60?

Anastrazole appeared to be especially potent for post-menopausal women under 60 years of age:

- Anastrozole (Arimidex)
94.9% of the women had no recurrence

- Tamoxifen
88.2% of the women had no recurrence

For women older than 60, anastrazole (Arimidex) and tamoxifen were equally effective at reducing DCIS recurrence risk. The researchers said they didn't have a good explanation for why anastrozole and tamoxifen offered equal benefits to women older than 60 (as opposed to the post-menopausal women under 60, for whom anastrazole provided more benefit than did tamoxifen).

DCIS

Into the future: HER2 and prognosis

Her2 overexpression may predict an increased risk of local (in-breast) recurrence. Radiation therapy reduces local failure rates for HER2-positive DCIS. Here are the results (with a median followup of 7.6 years) from the European Institute of Oncology in which roughly a third of patients with DCIS had HER2 overexpression:

> The adjusted risk of an DCIS breast cancer recurrence was higher in the HER2-positive group than in the HER2-negative group, by a factor of 1.59. This study did not support the premise that HER2-overexpression in primary DCIS is of any major importance for tumor progression toward *invasive* breast cancer.

HER2 testing not routine for DCIS
While we do not routinely test DCIS for HER2, there is an an ongoing trial (NSABP B-43) randomizing patients to adding the anti-HER2 drug Herceptin (trastuzumab) or not to conventional surgery and radiation therapy of patients whose DCIS overexpresses HER2.

High-risk DCIS treated with breast-conserving surgery and radiation therapy has a low risk of local recurrence. The addition of a costly drug such as trastazumab (Herceptin) in order to reduce this small risk further is very unlikely to be cost-effective and could be considered overtreatment of a non-fatal disease that is sufficiently managed with current management approaches.

DCIS

Into the future: Genomics

Oncotype DX DCIS is a 12-panel gene test with a scoring system that categorizes ductal carcinoma *in situ* as low, intermediate, or high risk for local recurrence over the 10 years following treatment with breast-conserving surgery alone. A large population-based study presented at the 2014 San Antonio Breast Cancer Symposium validated this gene test in a diverse population of women with DCIS.

Should you have OncoType DX testing for DCIS?

This test needs further study and is *not* yet part of standard practice. However, if you and your doctor agree that the test is right for you, you will likely want to find out if the test is covered by your insurance. During surgery, your doctor will remove and preserve a small amount of tumor. The pathologist will send sections of the tumor to Genomic Health to generate a DCIS Score™ result, which is then reported to your doctor. The DCIS Score results tell the likelihood or possibility of the cancer returning in the same breast as either a DCIS tumor or as an invasive breast cancer tumor:

Risk group	Local recurrence
Low	13%
Intermediate	**28%**
High	**33%**

OncoType DX produces the DCIS Score™ result, a number between 0 and 100. Women with lower DCIS Score results have a lower risk of their DCIS returning as DCIS or as an invasive tumor. A higher DCIS Score result means that there is a greater chance of the cancer returning.

Microinvasion

Prognosis: Excellent

Microinvasive breast carcinoma is defined as invasive carcinoma of the breast with no invasive focus measuring more than 1 millimeter. It is often found in the setting of ductal carcinoma *in situ* (DCIS), and some refer to it as DCIS with microinvasion. Data regarding the clinical significance of microinvasive carcinoma is limited, given it represents less than 1 percent of all cancers.

The prognosis for patients with microinvasive carcinoma is excellent, with 5-year survival chances ranging from 97 to 100%. In a series from Yale (USA) with a median follow-up of 8.5 years, there was no difference in the recurrence rate or 5-year survival odds when comparing patients with microinvasion and those with pure DCIS.

In-breast recurrence
The risk of a local recurrence following breast conserving- or mastectomy-based management appears to be small. Researchers from the Harvard-affiliated Brigham & Women's Hospital/Dana-Farber Cancer Institute have reported their experience. Here is the 5-year local recurrence rate for the patients having breast-conserving management for microinvasive carcinoma:

	Local recurrence
Breast-conserving management	4.2%

⚠ Close (2 mm or less) or involved (as opposed to negative or clear) surgical margins increased the risk of an in-breast recurrence after breast-conserving management or mastectomy by a whopping factor of 8.8-times! On the other hand, HER-2 overexpression was not associated with recurrence.

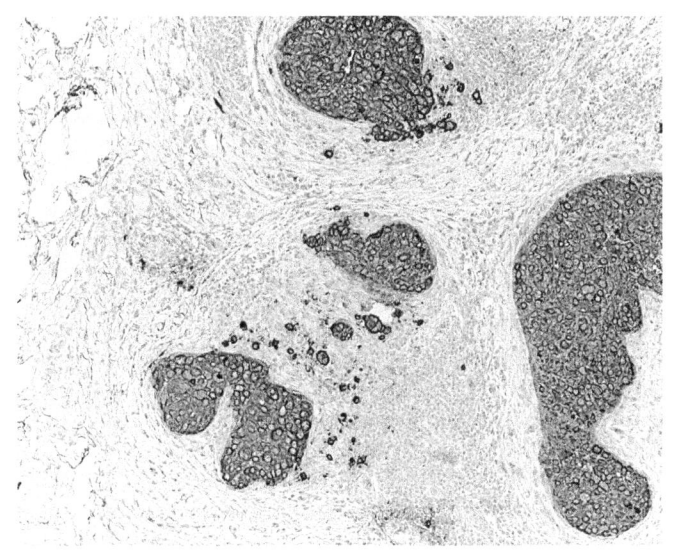

Microinvasive

Summary

Prognostic factors

- **Prognostic factors** provide information on outcomes, independent of treatment. In contrast, **predictive factors** provide information on the likelihood of a response to a given treatment. Some factors are both prognostic and predictive.

- **Stage (extent of cancer at diagnosis)** is a critical determinant of prognosis.

- **Lymphvascular (angiolymphatic) space invasion** (LVI) is a risk factor for local recurrence after breast-conserving management.

- **Both very younger and very old age** at diagnosis are associated with worse prognoses.

- **African-American women (as a group) have a worse prognosis,** compared with white and Asian women (even after controlling for disease characteristics at diagnosis).

- **Genomic assays** allow for the simultaneous measurement of thousands of genes, and have led to the identification of biology-based prognostic profiles that are in clinical use today. These assays incorporate important gene clusters relating to erstrogen receptor expression (the uminal cluster), HER2 expression, proliferation, and the basal gene cluster. **Breast cancer subtypes differ in prognosis.**

- **Local and/or regional recurrence prognostic factors** incude site of recurrence, volume of disease, and interval from original diagnosis to the time of recurrence.

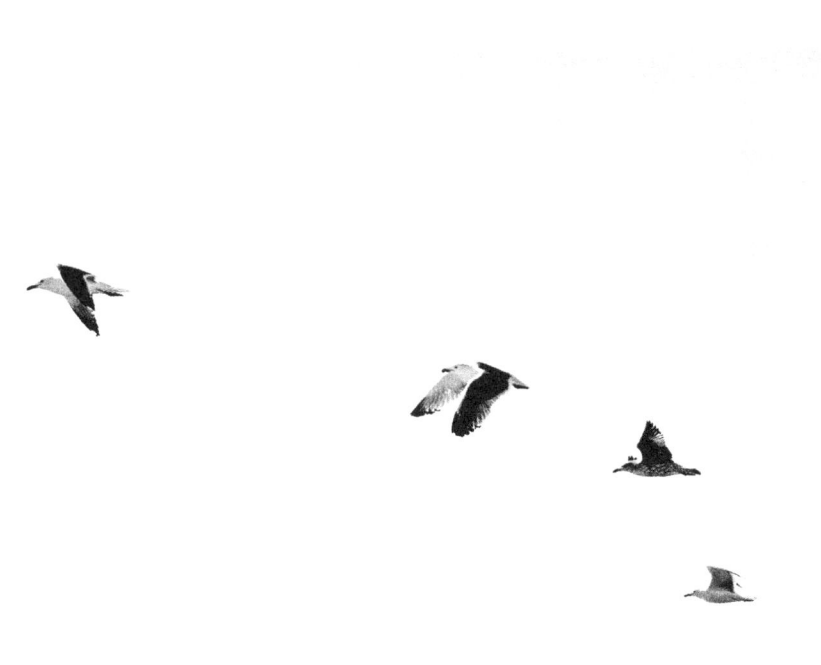

MANAGEMENT
BEFORE SURGERY

DCIS

Overview

Basics

Ductal carcinoma *in situ* (DCIS) is non-invasive. However, abnormal cells sometimes evolve to become invasive cancer over time. Left untreated, it is estimated that approximately 40 to 50 percent of DCIS cases may progress to invasive breast cancer. The diagnosis of DCIS increased dramatically following the introduction of screening mammograms, and now represents up to a quarter of all newly diagnosed breast cancer. In this chapter, we will review the maagement of DCIS.

Work-up

1) History and physical exam; 2) *diagnostic* mammograms of both breasts; 3) a review of the biopsy by a pathologist; and 4) determination of whether the DCIS has estrogen receptors (ER-positive or ER-negative). Genetic counseling is advised for individuals at high risk for hereditary breast cancer. Selected patients may have MRI of the breasts, although MRI has bot been shown to increase the likelihood of clear margins, or improve long-term outcomes.

Management

- Breast-conserving surgery ("lumpectomy") + radiation therapy
- Breast removal (mastectomy)
- Breast-conserving surgery

Breast treatment may be followed by consideration of anti-estrogen therapy such as tamoxifen pills (for pre- or postmenopausal women) or an aromatase inhibitor (for women who are after menopause). Follow-up is then a history and physical exam every 6 to 12 months for 5 years, then annually. Mammograms are done every 12 months (and 6 to 12 months after radiation therapy).

DCIS

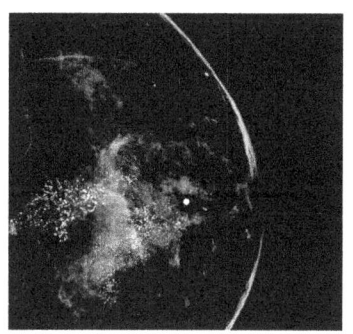

Imaging

Mammograms

Screening mammogram is the primary imaging tool for the early detection of breast cancer. The prototype of the mammography unit was developed in 1965. Two views are generally taken, one from top-down, and the other from side-to-side of the breast. Research suggests that 11 to 25 percent of cancers could be missed if only one view was obtained. A newer form of mammograms is known as tomosynthesis, or "3D" mammograms. A large study found that the addition of tomosynthesis to digital mammography resulted in a decrease in recall rates, and an increase in cancer detection rates.

We use *screening mammograms* for those with no clinical symptoms or findings on exam. On the other hand, a *diagnostic mammogram* is performed for patients who present with breast symptoms or have an abnormal clinical exam. The diagnostic mammogram is supervised by a radiologist, with images obtained to evaluate a specific abnormality. A spot compression view may be added, using focal compression to the area of interest in the breast using a small compression paddle. Magnification spot compression view can better characterize the shape and size of calcifications, or better characterize a mass.

Roughly 90 percent of women with DCIS have microcalcifications on mammography. DCIS accounts for 80 percent of breast cancer among those who presnt with calcifications on screening mammography. However, tomosynthesis did *not* improve detection rates for DCIS.

Ultrasound

Ultrasound uses sound waves to follow-up an abnormal mammogram. Ultrasound can provide more information about masses or asymmetry, and may distinguish a solid mass from a non-cancerous cyst. Ultrasound does not emit radiation.

DCIS

Imaging

MRI

The use of magnetic resonance imaging as sa screening tool for women at average risk is controversial. While its use for DCIS remains unclear, the test may help to determine the extent of DCIS and to identify disease theat is scattered in the breast (muticentric DCIS) or find cancer in the opposite (contralateral) breast. Many centers do not use MRI for DCIS: While MRI is quite good at finding DCIS, its use is linked to a high risk of false alarms, known as false positives.

Should everyone with ductal carcinoma *in situ* have a breast MRI? About one third of surgeons in the United States will order an MRI for women with DCIS. Yet routine use of MRI before or after surgery in women with DCIS may not be a sound clinical strategy: It does *not* appear to improve long-term outcomes. Researchers at Memorial Sloan Ketterin Cancer Center (New York City) identified 2321 women who had undergone lumpectomy for DCIS between 1997 and 2010. Of these patients, 596 received an MRI either before or immediately after surgery and 1725 did not.

After 8 years, local recurrence rates were *not* significantly different between the MRI and no-MRI groups (14.6% vs 10.2%). Even after controlling for nine patient variables (including such as age, menopausal status, family history, and use of radiation or endocrine therapy), there was no significant difference in the risk of local recurrence. This multivariable analysis is important because women who undergo MRI will typically have a higher risk profile. Finally, contralateral (the other) breast cancer rates in the MRI and no-MRI groups were the same: Contralateral breast cancer rates in the MRI and no-MRI groups were the same at 5 years (3.5% vs 3.5%) and similar at 8 years (3.5% vs 5.1%). To me, this does not mean that no patient with DCIS should have an MRI; rather, I think we don't have high-level evidence to advocate for its *routine* use for patients with ductal carcinoma *in situ*.

DCIS

Biopsy types

Core needle biopsy

An abnormality may be evaluated by a core tissue sampling. When possible, this is preferred to alternatives such as removal of the lesion (excisional biopsy). The core biopsy is done with image guidance.

Wire localization excisional biopsy

For those who are not candidates for non-surgical approaches (such as a core biopsy) to establish the diagnosis, an alternative is a so-called wire localization excisional biopsy. This technique involves the placement of a very thin wire. This allows your surgeon to localize the tissue that needs to be removed. The wire is placed in the radiology department of a hospital or surgery center where your breast biopsy ("lumpectomy') is to be performed.

You are awake for the placement of the very fine wire, but the radiologist injects a local anesthetic to numb the breast before placement. You may experience a bit of a sting from the anesthetic needle, but most patients feel much more comfortable as the anesthetic begins to act. Images are taken of your breast. The radiologist then inserts a very fine needle to target the breast abnormality. The aim is to rest the tip of the needle at the location of the abnormality. A slender wire is threaded down through the needle and the needle is then removed (with the wire left in place). It is not unusual to feel pressure or a pulling sensation during the wire placement. Another mammogram is done to ensure that the wire is in just the right spot, and then the wire is secured in place with tape or a bandage. Now you are ready for your surgery.

What entities could potentially be mistaken for DCIS? Atypical ductal hyperplasia (ADH), microinvasive carcinoma, and lobular carcinoma *in situ* (LCIS) all can look like DCIS. The odds that a seemingly pure DCIS on a core needle biopsy will be associated with an invasive cancer at surgery is on the order of 25%.

Genes

Management: Genetic counseling

I want to make a brief detour to talk a bit about genetic counseling, as it can affect your decision regarding which type of breast surgery to pursue. We will go in more detail in a later chapter. Might you be a candidate for genetic testing?

You have breast cancer and ...	• you have have a known mutation (in the family) of a gene that increases cancer risk • you are 50 or under • you are 60 or under with ER/PR/HER2 negative breast cancer • you have 2 breast cancers* • you are of Ashkenazi Jewish descent • you are male • you have 1+ close blood relatives with breast cancer found at 50 years or younger (or with ovarian, fallopian, or primary peritoneal cancer); 2 or more close blood relatives with breast, pancreas and/or prostate cancer (Gleason score 7 or higher)
You have a personal history of **ovarian cancer**	

Other criteria include a personal and/or family history of at least three of the following:

- Breast, pancreas, prostate (Gleason score 7+), diffuse stomach (gastric), colon, endometrial, thyroid, or kidney cancer, melanoma, sarcoma, adrenocortical carcinoma, brain tumors, or leukemia

- Skin problems consistent with Cowden syndrome

- Macrocephaly, hamartomatous polyps of the gastrointestinal tract

---

* bilateral disease or at least two separate cancers in the same breast

BRCA

Breast cancer genes (basics)

Patients at high risk for having hereditary (inherited) breast cancer should receive **genetics counseling.** Approximately 5% to 10% of breast cancer patients have an inherited genetic mutation related to their cancer. The most common gene mutations (mistakes) associated with breast cancer are ones in tumor suppression genes BRCA1 and BRCA2 (BReast CAncer genes #1 and #2). You may recall that the actress Angelina Jolie had a BRCA mutation.

Breast cancer risk
About 12 percent of women in the general population will develop breast cancer during their lives. By contrast, 72 percent of women who inherit a harmful BRCA1 mutation and around 69 percent of women who inherit a harmful BRCA2 mutation will develop breast cancer by 80 years of age. In addition, breast cancer incidence was noted to rise in early adulthood until 30 to 40 years for BRCA1 carriers, and until 40 to 50 years for BRCA2 carriers, after which it plateaued at 20 to 30 per 1000 person years until at least age 80. BRCA1 carriers are more likely to develop a so-called triple negative breast cancer, an especially aggressive form of the disease.

Ovarian cancer risk
About 1.3 percent of women in the general population will develop ovarian cancer sometime during their lives. By contrast, 44 percent of women who inherit a harmful BRCA1 mutation (and 17 percent of women who inherit a harmful BRCA2 mutation) will develop ovarian cancer by age 70 years.

BRCA mutations increase risk of other cancers, too
The incidence may increase for cancer of the opposite breast, colon (BRCA1; amount uncertain), male prostate cancer (BRCA2 may increase risk 5- to 9-fold; the magnitude of increase for BRCA1 carriers is not well-understood), and pancreas cancer (BRCA1 unclear; BRCA2 5 percent, compared to 1.5 percent in the general population). We are learning about the risk of stomach and biliary cancer (BRCA2), skin or uveal (eye) melanoma for those with BRCA2 mutations, fallopian tube cancer (lifetime risk about 0.6 percent) uterine papillary serious carcinoma, and others.

Inherited mutations

A special note for those with a BRCA mutation

Many women with a harmful BRCA1 or BRCA2 mutation who develop breast cancer in one breast choose a bilateral (double) mastectomy, even if they would otherwise be candidates for breast-conserving surgery.

And the ovaries, too?

We do not have very effective tools for ovarian cancer screening. You may also wish to consider removing your ovaries and fallopian tubes in a procedure known as a bilateral salpingo-oophorectomy (BSO), depending on where you are in your life and whether you wish to have biological children. Some women choose to delay the procedure until age 40 to 45. I recommend a referral to a gynecologic oncologist for a discussion about this surgery. The surgery appears to not only reduce the risk of ovarian cancer among BRCA mutation carriers, but also decreases the risk of dying of the disease.

Other risk-reducing surgery?

Risk-reducing removal of the ovaries and fallopian tubes is the procedure of choice, with a removal of the uterus (hysterectomy) not routinely recommended. I am unaware of national guideines pointing to the taking of the uterus, even though there may be a small increase in the incidence of uterus cancer among BRCA mutation carriers. There is controversy about removing only the fallopian tubes, for those who want to keep their ovaries for some time. Alas, we do not have high-level evidence from clinical trials to support this limited approach.

Hormone replacement (HRT)

Prior to using HRT to manage menopausal symptoms in BRCA carriers who have had a risk-reducing removal of their ovaries and fallopian tubes, there should be a shared decision-making process including counseling about non-hormonal options and our lack of high-level evidence regarding hormone replacement therapy for carriers of BRCA mutations. Similarly, we lack high-level evidence regarding the use of vaginal estrogen therapy for carriers.

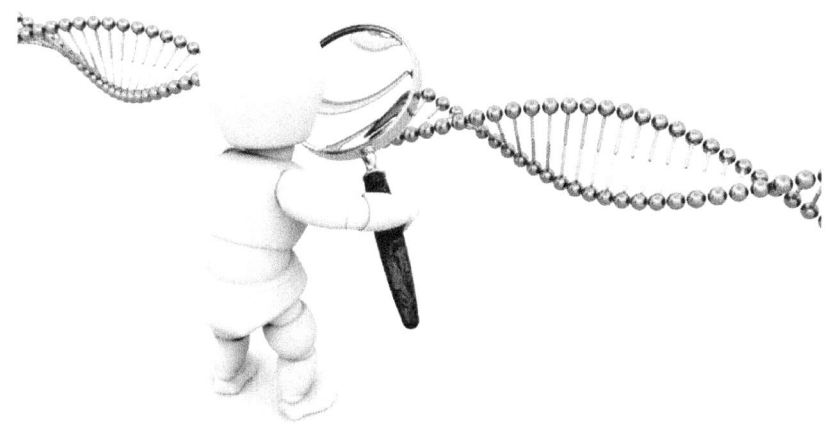

Many women with a harmful **BRCA1 or BRCA2** mutation who develop breast cancer in one breast choose a bilateral (double) mastectomy, even if they would otherwise be candidates for breast-conserving surgery.

DCIS

Paget disease of the nipple

Paget disease of the breast (also known as Paget disease of the nipple and mammary Paget disease) is a rare type of cancer involving the skin of the nipple and often the darker circle of skin around it (areola). Most people with Paget disease of the breast also have one or more tumors inside the same breast. A biopsy of the nipple abnormality is required to diagnose Paget disease of the breast. Several types of biopsy are available, including the following:

- *Surface biopsy*
  A glass slide (or other tool) igently scrape cells from the skin.
- *Shave biopsy*
  A razor-like tool removes the skin's top layer.
- *Punch biopsy*
  A circular cutting tool (a punch) removes a disk-shaped piece of tissue.
- *Wedge biopsy*
  A scalpel is used to remove a small wedge of tissue.

Less commonly, the surgeon may remove the entire nipple. A pathologist then examines the cells under a microscope to make a diagnosis. It is not uncommon for individuals with Paget disease of the nipple to simultaneously have a separate cancer in the same breast. Thus the imaging and physical exam are critical. In fact, as many as 50 percent of patients with Paget disease of the nipple may have an underlying mass in the breast that can be felt. (1, 2).

Here are some the features for which the pathologist looks to make the diagnosis of Paget disease: 1) intraepithelial (within the layer of cells that forms the surface or lining the nipple) population of large, atypical (Paget) cells; 2) large nuclei, with prominent nucleoli (small dense spherical structures in the nucleus of a cell during interphase part of the cell life cycle); 3) an underlying *in situ* or invasive breast carcinoma is commonly present.

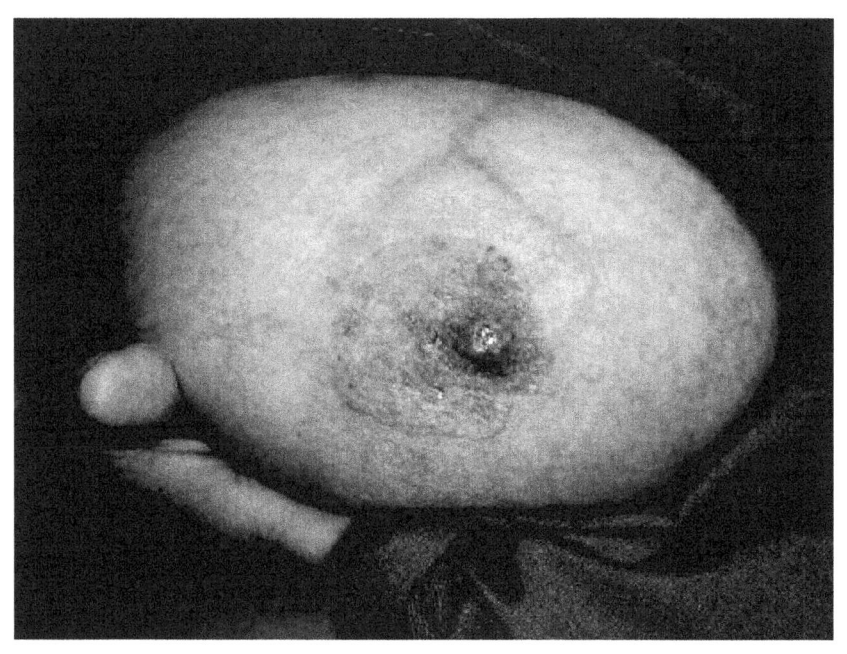

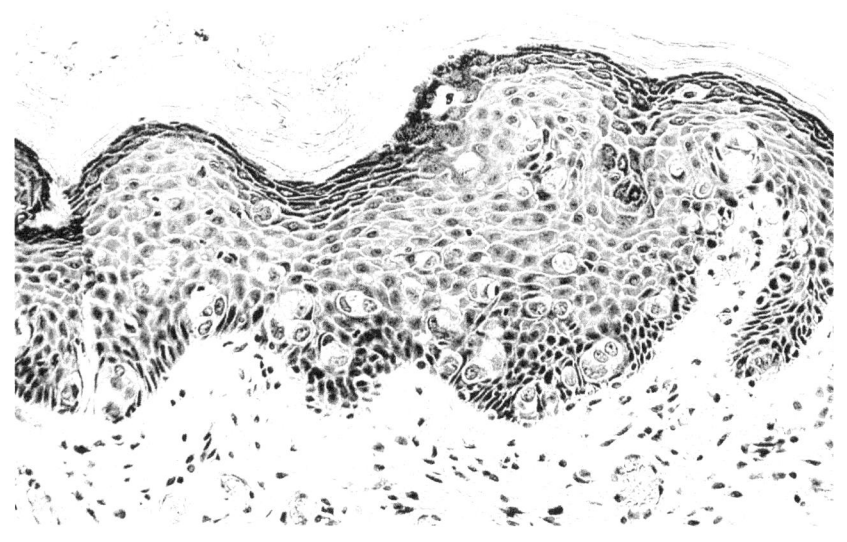

MANAGEMENT
SURGERY

DCIS

Management

Goals

The term ductal carcinoma *in situ* (DCIS) of the breast really refers to a group of diseases with various potential behaviors. All DCIS types have this in common: They are confined to the breast ducts, and in their pure form cannot spread or threaten your life. *In situ* means "remaining in place." Our management goal is to prevent the development of invasive breast cancer. Potential tools include surgery, radiation therapy, and anti-estrogen (endocrine) therapy.

Surgery

We begin with surgery. Women with DCIS may have local (breast) treatment with a mastectomy or with a breast-conserving approach. Breast conserving management consists of a lumpectomy (wide excision; partial mastectomy), typically followed by radiation therapy. Let's look at these approaches:

> **Mastectomy versus lumpectomy**
> Both are reasonable options for most women with small volume, DCIS that is confined to a single area of the breast. If you meet the criteria for a lumpectomy, the surgery choice is a personal one. A mastectomy is excellent long-term disease-specific survival (and local control). Still, mastectomy may be overly aggressive surgery for the majority of women with DCIS. While a lumpectomy is generally better tolerated, there is a higher chance of a local (in-breast) recurrence with a breast-conserving approach.
>
> The 20-year odds of surviving appear to be similar (about 97% overall) when comparing mastectomy with lumpectomy-based approaches. However, there is a higher local recurrence rate (for example, 3.3 percent versus 1.3 percent in one series) with breast-conserving management.

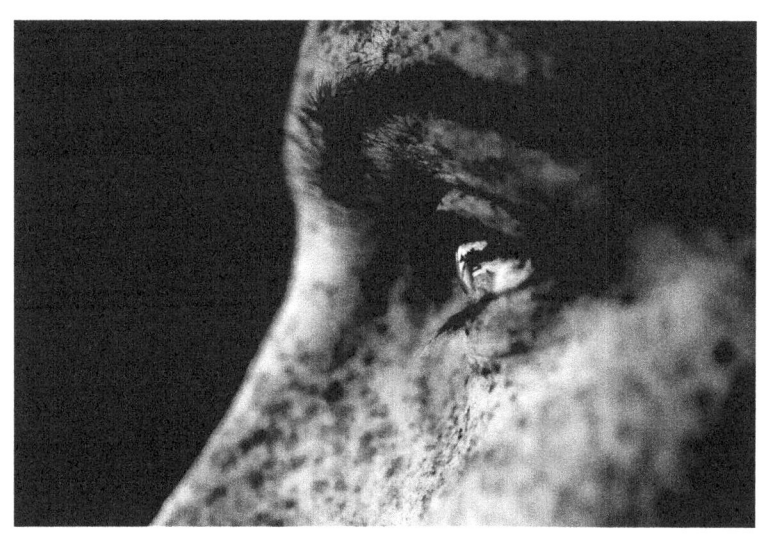
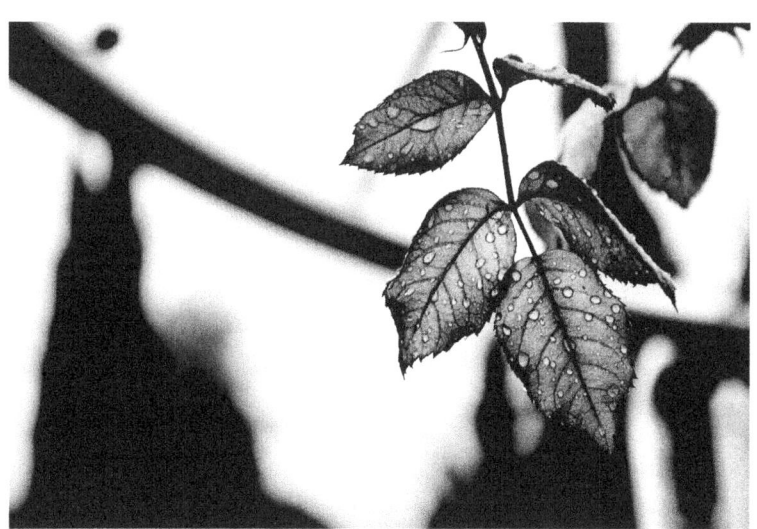

Criteria for breast conserving surgery

The data suggests breast conserving management for DCIS results in a low rate of in-breast recurrence with a favorable side effect profile. Still, mastectomy is a reasonable alternative approach for many women. To be a candidate for breast conservation, there are certain criteria that must be met:

- *Limited*

  The DCIS should be limited to one quadrant or section of the breast. If it is multicentric (that is, in breast locations far apart from one another), a mastectomy is indicated. The finding of multiple lesions in close proximity to one another is not necessarily mean you cannot have breast conserving surgery.

- *Reasonable cosmesis*

  A resection would yield a cosmetic outcome acceptable to you.

- *Margins, margins, margins*

  A reasonable cancer-free zone (clear or negative margins) around the DCIS can be achieved. Margin status is an important factor for achieving local (in-breast) control. Re-resection(s) may be performed in an effort to obtain clear (negative) margins for those desiring breast-conserving management.

Mastectomy

If these criteria are *not* met, a mastectomy is usually the preferred management approach. Mastectomy is curative for over 98 percent of patients with DCIS. Some women who have a mastectomy for the breast with the DCIS will elect to remove the other breast as a risk-reducing maneuver (prophylactic contralateral mastectomy). I am unaware of an associated survival benefit for doing so, however. Other women choose to use endocrine therapy (such as tamoxifen or aromatase inhibitor pills) as a risk-reducing maneuver.

While the removal of axillary (underarm) nodes is not indicated for most women with DCIS, those undergoing a mastectomy for DCIS may benefit from a so-called sentinely lymph node biopsy. This check of a node is not mandatory, but some surgeons prefer to do it: After a total mastectomy, the lymphatic drainage is permanently changed, rendering it impossible to perform an accurate sentinel node biopsy if we discover you actually had invasive cancer in the removed breast tissue.

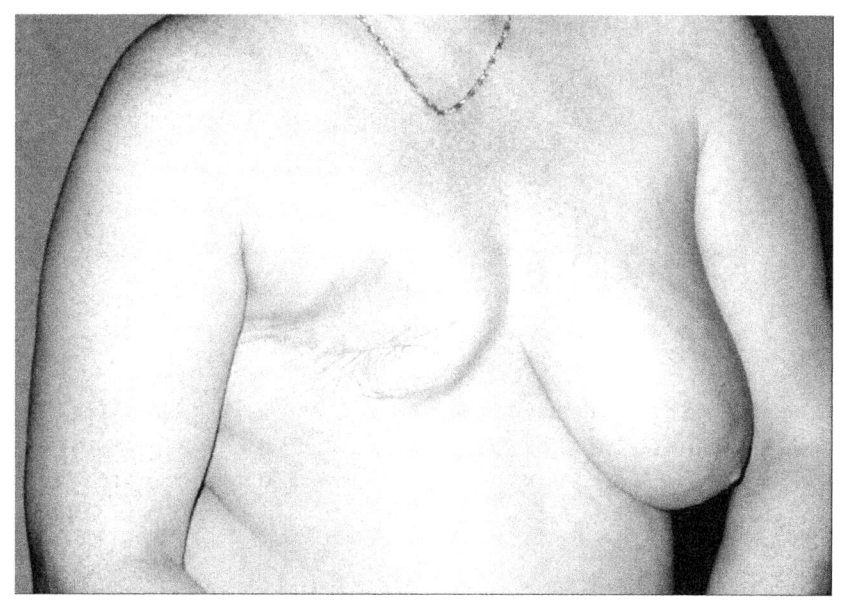

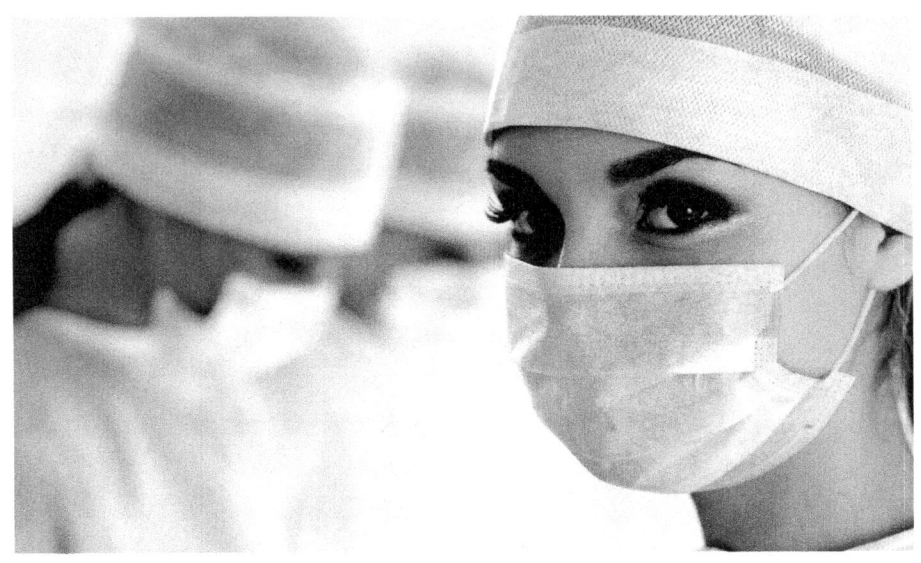

Surgery: Logistics

Preop

If your cancer cannot be felt or seen, you will need a procedure before surgery to mark the target tumor using imaging such as a mammogram. A care provider may also draw marks (using a felt-tip marker, for example) on your breast that show where the incision will be made.

You are then taken to the anesthesia room, where a nurse inserts an intravenous (IV) line into your hand or arm, taping it into place. While many patients who have a lumpectomy have a local numbing anesthesia, some have general anesthesia. General anesthesia is typically used if you will also have lymph nodes removed, for example with a simple mastectomy.

A lumpectomy surgery usually lasts about 30 to 45 minutes. Your surgeon will likely use an electric scalpel that uses heat to reduce bleeding. The scar is often (but not always) curved, following your breast's natural curves. The tumor is removed, along with a small surrounding rim of normal-appearing breast tissue. With a lumpectomy, most patient do not need a drain placed in the breast or axilla. At the end of the operation, your surgeon will stitch the incision closed and cover the wound.

Nodes

Management: Sentinel node(s)

Complications

We have an abundance of evidence showing the sentinel lymph node biopsy to be associated with fewer side effects than the more invasive axillary lymph node dissection. For appropriately selected patients, the use of the sentinel lymph node mapping does *not* compromise your survival or increase your risk of a recurrence in the axilla. Here are the results of 5611 patients enrolled in the National Surgical Adjuvant Breast and Bowel Project (NSABP) B-32 study.

	Sentinel	**Axillary dissection**
Limb swelling	8%	14%
Numbness	8%	31%
Arm movement deficits	13%	19%
Seroma	Not available	

A meta-analysis (a study of a collection of 7 published reports) comparing an axillary lymph node dissection versus a sentinel lymph node biopsy showed a reduction in risk of infection, seroma, arm swelling, and numbness among patients who had the sentinel node procedure. These results suggest that the sentinel node mapping is the new standard for staging the vast majority of patients early breast cancer. It is not standard to perform a lymph node sampling for those with ductal carcinoma *in situ,* unless it is done as a part of a mastectomy.

Remember: Most patients with DCIS do *not* need a sampling of the axillary (underarm) lymph nodes. It is not uncommon to have a sentinel node procedure with a mastectomy for DCIS, however, as there is a chance that the pathologist will find an invasive component in the removed material, and we typically would need to check a lymph node if that were the case.

DCIS

Surgery

Most patients who are given both options prefer the less invasive, breast-conserving management approach. How do you choose?

- *Do I want to keep my breast?*
If you are deemed an appropriate candidate, you may wish to consider lumpectomy (typically followed by radiation therapy).

- *Am I anxious about cancer coming back in the breast?*
If breast removal would significantly reduce your anxiety about an in-breast recurrence (and if you understand that a mastectomy does not improve your survival chances, as compared to a breast-conserving approach), you may wish to consider a mastectomy. While there are no long-term differences in your odds for survival, there is a higher risk of a local recurrence after a lumpectomy, compared to after a mastectomy..

- *Are you okay with receiving radiation therapy?*
Radiation therapy courses vary in length, but are often composed of 15 minute appointments, Monday through Friday for three to four weeks (and occasionally up to seven weeks). Partial breast approaches can be faster; for example, twice a day radiation therapy for 5 days.

The overwhelming majority of patients having a mastectomy for DCIS do *not* need radiation therapy, unless the lymph nodes are involved or the margins are under a millimeter.

- *Does having a mastectomy mean I won't need chemo?*
Chemotherapy is *not* used for DCIS, irrespective of the surgery type.

- *My tumor is fairly large. Must I have a mastectomy?*
Selected patients who have tumors that are large (relative to the breast) or extensively throughout the breast (multicentric or diffuse concerning calcifications) typically need a breast removal (mastectomy).

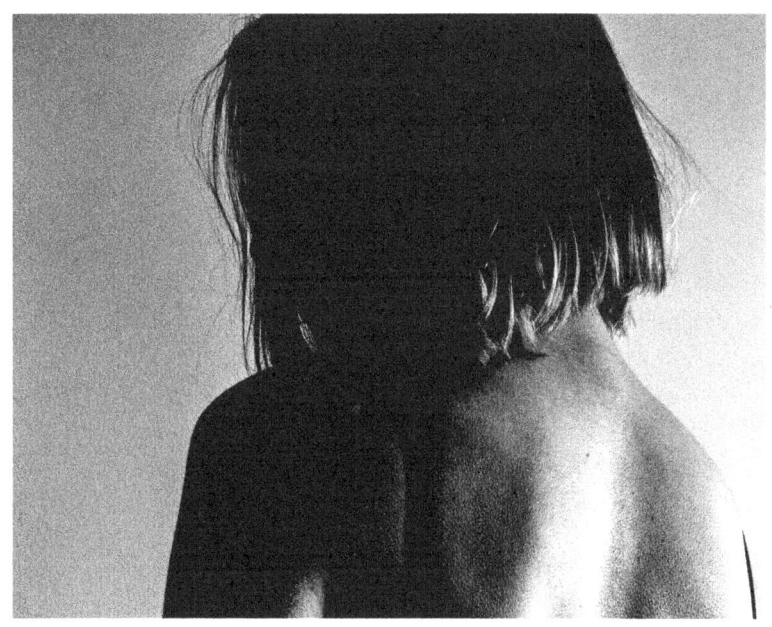

After mastectomy: Reconstruction

Breast reconstruction should be available to those women undergoing mastectomy. Immediate reconstruction for many women can make the prospect of losing a breast easier to accept, but not all patients are candidates for immediate reconstruction. Some women may decline or defer reconstruction because of personal preference.

The autologous tissue-based techniques generally tolerate postoperative RT well. Implant-based reconstruction can result in an unfavourable aesthetic outcome, following postoperative RT. Skin-sparing mastectomy allows the skin envelope to be conserved for use in the breast reconstruction.

DCIS

Management: Care after surgery

You will be moved to the recovery room, where care providers monitor your heart rate, blood pressure, and temperature. Most patients having a lumpectomy leave the same day, unless lymph nodes are removed. As you recover at home, you may need to:

- **Take pain medication**

Many patients have the prescription filled on their way home. While you may or may not need the pain medicine, it is wise to have it available, although I would avoid the use of the narcotic pain medicine if possible..

- **Take care of a bandage.**

Your surgeon or valued care team member should give you instructions. On occasion, the surgeon will ask you to wait until your first follow-up visit, at which time the bandage (dressing) may be removed.

- **Stitches and staples**

Stitches (sutures) are typically used, and dissolve over time. It is not rare to see the end of the stitch (suture) sticking out of the incision like a whisker. If this is the case, your surgeon can remove it. Staples are not common, but if used, they are removed during your first post-operative follow-up visit.

- **Consider a good support or sports bra.**

This may reduce movement that can cause pain. Many with larger breasts prefer to sleep on the side that has not been operated upon, sometimes with the healing breast supported by a pillow in front of them.

- **Consider sponge baths until your doctor removes your drains and/or stitches (sutures)**

Sponge baths may prove refreshing until your doctor gives you the okay for showers or baths.

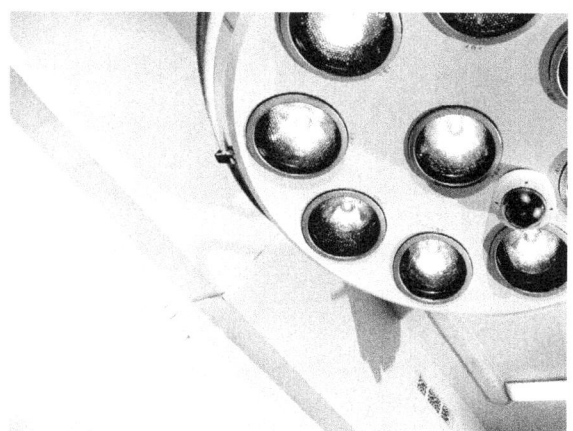

Are there other things I can do following a lumpectomy?

- **Watch for infection**
Ask your care providers about symptoms.

- **Rest**
You may feel tired after surgery, so try to get enough rest. Most patients get back into their normal routine after several days.

- **Arm exercises**
Your surgeon, physical therapist, or other care team member may show you an exercise routine to reduce the probability of arm and shoulder stiffness after the surgery. Typically, you may begin light arm exercises the day after surgery, but some exercises should not be done while drains are in place. Please ask your surgeon about a routine that is appropriate for you.

Breast conserving surgery: Intermediate-term symptoms

Many patient report sensitivity to touch, some itchiness, or fleeting sharp, shooting pains. These symptoms typically resolve over time. If the discomfort persists, check with your care providers to see if you might be a candidate to take medicines such as acetaminophen or ibuprofen. Uncommonly, stronger pain medicines are needed.

DCIS

Surgery

Margins

The margin width (distance between the edge of the DCIS and the nearest inked margin) reflects the completeness of surgical removal of the DCIS, and is an important predictor of local recurrence. This is especially true for those who opt to avoid radiation therapy. We characterize the margins as:

- *Negative ("clean", "not involved" or "clear")*
The margins don't contain cancer cells: There is only normal tissue at the edges of the tissue removed from the breast. No additional DCIS surgery is typically needed.

- *Positive ("involved") margins*
The margins contain cancer cells. More surgery is typically recommended to get clear margins. On occasion, it is not possible or necessary to get clear margins due to location (for example, if it is at the chest wall).

- *Close margins*
DCIS approaches, but doesn't touch the edge of the breast tissue removed. More surgery may or may not be needed.

To further ensure the tumor has been removed, the excised breast tissue may be X-rayed ("specimen radiograph"). This may be especially useful when microcalcifications were found on a mammogram and are related to the cancer. Depending on the X-ray results, more tissue may be removed at surgery (immediate re-excision). After surgery, selected patients *may* have a mammogram of the affected breast, if there is any concern that concerning disease (calcifications) have been left behind. This is especially true if the calcifications are extensive before surgery, approach the edge of the surgical specimen, or the surgical margins are not completely clear.

Clear margins are important for local control

For women with ductal carcinoma *in situ* (DCIS) who are treated with breast-conserving surgery, margin status is recognized as one of the most important predictors of local recurrence regardless of whether radiation therapy is given after surgery. A recent meta-analysis (analysis of a collection of studies) showed:

- *Positive (involved) margins:* In-breast relapse is 2.25 times higher

- *Negative (uninvolved) margins:* In-breast relapse is lower with margins larger than 10 mm, compared to a negative margin larger than 2 mm

Let's look in graphic form at the predicted probabilities of an in-breast re-currence, stratified by margin threshold and treatment (RT is radiation therapy):

	Positive	Margin threshold			
		0 mm	2 mm	5 mm	10 mm
Lumpectomy + RT	**20%**	10%	9%	11%	**4%**
Lumpectomy alone	**35%**	20%	17%	20%	**9%**

There has been a lack of consensus about what constitutes an optimal cancer-free or "negative" margin for ductal carcinoma *in situ*, and as result, about historically one in three DCIS surgeries have been repeated to obtain better margins. After evaluating a new meta-analysis (collection of studies), **a consensus panel concluded that 2 millimeters (mm) is optimal:** Wider margins were not associated with a lower in-breast recurrence rate, and margins less than this led to a higher probability of an in-breast recurrence. The 2 millimeter margin (while often preferred) is not required, however, especially for those receiving radiation therapy.

⚠️ **Clear surgical margins** should be obtained for DCIS patients after breast conserving surgery, regardless of whether radiation therapy is to be given. Within cosmetic constraint, surgeons should attempt to achieve negative margins as wide as reasonably achievable in their first attempt.

MANAGEMENT
RADIATION

DCIS

Treatment

Radiation therapy (RT)

Breast conserving surgery ("lumpectomy") with the achievement of clear margins is commonly followed by radiation therapy (RT). Patients at very low risk may opt to decline radiation therapy, as may those with other medical problems or limited life expectancy. RT reduces the risk of local invasive and non-invasive recurrences. Randomized trials have shown **RT applied after surgery reduces the risk of an in-breast tumor recurrence by 50 percent or more,** compared with excision alone. Let's look at one of the best studies comparing radiation therapy versus surgery with no radiation therapy (15 year results):

National Surgical Breast and Bowel Project (NSABP) Trial B-17

	RT	No RT
• In-breast *invasive* recurrence	9%	**19%**
• Survival	83%	84%

Radiation therapy reduces recurrence risk by half

A systematic review of radiation therapy after surgery for DCIS incuded four randomized controlled trials involving 3925 women. Radiation therapy reduced the risk of in-breast recurrence by half. All subgroups (margin status, age, and grade) benefited from the addition of radiation therapy.

Nine women required treatment with radiotherapy to prevent one in-breast recurrence. Deaths from vascular disease, lung toxicity, and second cancers were low and not significantly higher for women who received radiation therapy. The authors concluded that radiation therapy was beneficial for for all clinically relevant subgroups.

Radiation therapy or no RT: Long-term results

The SweDCIS (Swedish Ductal Carcinoma in Situ) trial was set up in 1987 to study the value of radiation therapy (RT) after breast-conserving surgery for breast ductal carcinoma *in situ* (DCIS). Here are the findings at the 20 year follow-up mark:

- Breast cancer–specific death
  Radiation therapy had no effect.
- Overall survival
  Radiation therapy had no effect.
- Half of recurrences were *in situ*, and half invasive breast cancer.
- Younger women had a relatively higher risk of local relapse.
- **Radiation therapy reduced the risk of *in situ* recurrences for all age groups,** whereas radiation therapy reduced the chances of an *invasive* local recurrence only for women 52 or older.

What you need to know

The Swedish researchers concluded that the use of radiation therapy (after lumpectomy) is supported by 20-year follow-up results. Long-term results have been presented for three similar studies randomly assigning patients to radiation therapy or not after breast conserving surgery for primary ductal carcinoma *in situ*. These studies found that **radiation therapy led to an absolute reduced risk of in breast recurrence of 10% after 15 years,** and the effect appears similar for *in situ* and invasive breast events. No effect on breast cancer survival was reported in any of the studies: Radiation therapy improves local (in-breast) control, but has no effects on your odds for survival.

"Good risk" DCIS

The Radiation Therapy Oncology Group 98-04 study identified so-called good-risk patients with DCIS; more specifically, theses patients had DCIS that was detected by screening mammogram, was low- or intermediate-grade, measured less than 2.5 centimeters, and jave margins of 3 millimeters or greater. In this good risk subset of patients with DCIS, after a median follow-up of 7 years, **the in-breast recurrence rate was significantly decreased by the addition of radiation therapy (7 percent versus 1 percent).**

DCIS

Treatment

Radiation therapy (RT)

Not all women who have had a lumpectomy for DCIS need radiation therapy, but RT can meaningfully lower your risk of an in-breast recurrence: The goal is to kill any DCIS cells that might be left in the breast after breast-preserving surgery (Radiation therapy is rarely needed after a mastectomy for DCIS). However, radiation therapy does not improve your odds for long-term survival. If radiation therapy is being considered, you will be referred to a radiation oncologist. The first step is a consultation, a meeting in which you will review the pros and cons of RT, alternatives to it, and logistics.

Am I a candidate for radiation therapy?

Some women with DCIS are not candidates for radiation therapy. For example, being pregnant or having certain health conditions can make radiation therapy risks higher. The latter include active scleroderma or lupus. Unfortunately, these disorders can cause harm to normal tissue during and after radiation therapy. In addition, if you have had radiation therapy to the same breast (or same general region of the chest area), you may not be a candidate for breast radiation therapy.

Simulation for external beam radiation therapy

If you opt for radiation therapy, you need to first have a treatment planning session (simulation). Here, the radiation oncology physician and a simulation therapist map out the target. Typically, you have a CT scan of your breast region, with no contrast administered by vein or mouth. You are placed on your back (supine) on a hard flat table, arms overhead. Many patients appreciate some support placed behind their knees. During the planning session, the radiation simulation therapist will pit small marks (about the size of a pinhead) on your skin, as these can help optimize targeting for each of the daily radiation treatments. The marks are commonly permanent tattoos.

Radiation treatment planning: Special considerations for left side

If radiation hits your heart, it may be injured. Typically, we use tangential fields, with the patient having arms over head, and the heart does not receive significant dose. If your treatment will be targeting the left breast, you may be asked to hold your breath (for short periods of time) during the planning session. This is one way to minimize radiation exposure to the heart: Deep inspirations typicaly causes the heart to fall backwards, out of the the radiation field. Not everyone can have (or needs) this innovative approach. Some cannot hold their breath consistently for the required time, and many radiation therapy centers don't have the necessary technology.

Each daily (Monday through Friday) radiation therapy session lasts about 20 minutes. Treatment is typically given for 3-7 weeks. The schedule of radiation sessions varies from person to person, depending on factors such as margin status, life expectancy, and body habitus.

Radiation dose: To boost or not to boost

Radiation therapy is most commonly delivered to the whole breast, for example over approximately 3 or 5 weeks. After the whole breast treatment, you may receive a supplemental dose of radiation targeting the area of the "lumpectomy," where the DCIS was located. This extra dose is called a "boost" and is typicaly aimed at a small volume. Most patients get their boost dose with a special form of external radiation called electrons. With electrons, we can regulate the depth of the radiation beam penetrance, for example by choosing a particular energy. A radiation "boost" to the tumor bed (the area from which the surgeon removed the DCIS) can yield a small, but statistically significant reduction in in-breast recurrence after a lumpectomy for ductal carcinoma *in situ*, retrospective study from the USA, Canada, and France has shown. Women who received the extra radiation therapy or boost had 15-year in-breast control rate of 91.6% compared with 88% for those who had lumpectomy and radiation therapy but no boost to the tumor bed.

Partial breast radiation therapy

Highly selected individuals may be candidates for more recently introduced radiation therapy techniques that target only the partial breast. These strategies include:

    1) Brachytherapy (MammoSite® is a well-known example).

    2) External beam radiation therapy

Management: Radiation after lumpectomy

Radiation type

Radiation therapy typically involves the delivery of beams made of either electrons or photons (X-rays). Electrons deposit most of their dose with a limited depth, determined largely by the electron energy selected. On the other hand, photons pass completely through tissues, so we angle the beams to cover the target breast or chest wall, in an effort to avoid critical organs such as the heart.

Radiation benefit

Whole breast external beam radiation therapy reduces the risk of a local or regional recurrence, and has been associated with a survival benefit as well. Prospective, randomized trials have shown a lowering of local recurrence chances with the incorporation of an additional boost dose of radiation therapy to the tumor bed.

Radiation treatment planning

Based on your cancer stage and other pathologic factors, we radiation oncologists define a target volume. For DCIS, the breast (or chest wall) is the primary target

Simulation is the planning session that you have prior to beginning radiation therapy. During simulation, your radiation oncologist will carefully define the radiation target, taking care to minimize risk to surrounding structures such as the heart and lung. There are two types of simulation: Virtual versus clinical simulation. For the former, we use low-dose CT scans (typically without contrast) to reconstruct high resolution digital films that can be used for planning. Clinical simulation requires that you are in the treatment position, while we do the actual planning. Most radiation therapy centers perform virtual simulation. For the simulation (treatment planning), some centers use a mold to hold you in the treatment position, as you lie on your back (supine). Markers may be placed to define the targets (for example, a wire may be placed around the breast and on the lumpectomy scar.

-

You are then imaged using a CT scanner, typically with 3 mm slice spacing through the desired treatment volume. With modern scanners, the entire procedure may be complete in under 30 minutes. Once the simulation is complete, a team that includes you doctor, dosimetrist, and others then design the fields, shaping it with metal leaves in the head of the treatment machine. A dosimetry plan shows the how the radiation dose is distributed. Once the fields, plan, and prescription are approved by your radiation oncologist, treatment can proceed.

Special situations

Patients with very large breast can represent a challenge for treatment planning, as the radiation therapy dose can be inhogeneous, creating so-called hot spots in areas such as the underarm region. On some occasions, we treat patients in the prone (lying on their abdomen, with the breast hanging through a hole in the positioning device) position, allowing the breast to fall away from critical structures such as the lung. Treatment of the internal mammary nodes (which lie next to the sternum, or breast bone) can also be challenging. Here, virtual simulation can allow your radiation oncologist to locate these lymph nodes with relative accuracy.

Management: Radiation after mastectomy

The vast majority of those with DCIS who have a mastectomy will not need radiation therapy. For the rare patient that does, the simulation (planning) techniques used to target the chest wall after mastectomy are similar to those we use for an intact breast. However, as the skin is usually an important target when radiation therapy is needed after mastectomy, you radiation oncologist may request that a material is placed on your skin during the treatment to ensure that full dose is delivered to the skin. This tissue equivalent material feels like rubber, and is known as *bolus*. The bolus allows the full dose to be delivered to the skin. The bolus may be placed daily, or every other day, and may be removed before you complete your treatment.

Radiation therapy

Management: Partial breast irradiation

A shorter course of radiation therapy can have great appeal. Accelerated partial breast irradiation (APBI) targets the tumor bed (the tumor location and not the whole breast), based in the fact that the majority of local recurrences occur in the vicinity of the primary tumor site. Accelerated partial breast irradiation might be considered an acceptable treatment option in patients with a low risk for local recurrence, for example those who are at least 50 years old with: unicentric, unifocal, node-negative, non-lobular breast cancer, up to 3 cm without the presence of extensive intraductal components or vascular invasion, and with negative margins, especially if they will receive adjuvant hormonal treatment. In the meantime, long-term results of several past and still on-going prospective randomised accelerated partial breast irradiation trials are eagerly awaited.

Accelerated partial breast irradiaton (APBI)

Accelerated partial breast irradiation uses focused radiation therapy to a limited portion of your breast. There are several options for the delivery of this localized form of radiation therapy:

- Conformal external beam radiation therapy (EBRT)
- Intensity modulated radiation therapy (IMRT)
- Brachytherapy (interstitial versus intracavitary)
- Intraoperative radiation therapy (IORT)

Conformal external beam radiation therapy

This 3-dimensional approach combines multiple radiation therapy fields to deliver dose to the tumor bed region (the zone from which the primary cancer was removed), while sparing the majority of your remaining breast tissue and solid organs. A typical dose is 35 to 38.5 Gy ("gray") in 10 treatmens (typically delivered twice per day, over a one week period).

Intensity modulated radiation therapy (IMRT)

For IMRT, we use a linear accelerator (treatment machine) to deliver highly focused small beams of radiation that allow the significant dose of radiation therapy to conform to the target tumor bed. The damage to surrounding tissue is less than for whole breast radiation. The use of IMRT for early breast cancer has been relatively limited, and requires clinical expertise and physics support.

Brachytherapy: Interstitial type

This specialized technique involves the placement of several small hollow catheters placed into the breast tissue that surrounds the tumor bed. High (or low) dose rate radioactive seeds are inserted into the catheters. The number of catheters used depends on the target size, and are removed after the procedure.

Brachytherapy: Intracavitary type

A radiation therapy delivery device is inserted into the tumor bed (where the cancer used to be) cavity at the time of your lumpectomy ("open technique") or several days after under ultrasound guidance ("closed technique") in an office setting. Some patients may have a cavity evaluation device placed at the time of surgery, with the device exchanged for the treatment one later.

Intraoperative radiation therapy

This form of RT reduces the entire dose into a single treatment administration, allowing surgery (lumpectomy) and radiation therapy to be completed in a single day. IORT permits the delivery of high doses of radiotherapy directly to the target tumor bed/surgical margins, while lowering dose to the skin and tissues just below the skin. IORT can lengthen the operative time, and we do not know the final surgical margins before the delivery of the radiation dose. We do not have long-term follow-up results.

Early results of (APBI) suggest that appropriately selected patients with early breast cancer may get local control rates comparable to those who have a course. We don't have long-term follow-up, and some recent studies hint at inferior cosmetic outcomes with APBI. The American Society for Radiation Oncology provides a consensus statement: Patients may be suitable for APBI if they are 60 and older, do not carry a BRCA gene mutation, and are treated with surgery for a unifocal T1, N0 estrogen receptor-positive cancer with uninvolved margins. The cancer should be ductal, and not associated with an extesive intraductal component or lobular carcinoma *in situ*.

Comparing the two approaches to radiation therapy (RT)

Accelerated partial breast radiation therapy appears to be nearly as effective as standard whole breast radiation therapy, at least with respect to reducing the risk of recurrence in the same breast for women with early stage breast cancer. We now have relatively long-term results from a large clinical trial examining the two approaches.

For this study, 4,216 women with stage 0, I, or II breast cancer who had a lumpectomy to remoev the cancer between 2005 and 2013 were randomly assigned to receive either whole breast radiation therapy (5 weeks to the whole breast, followed by a "boost" dose to the tumor bed) or accelerated partial breast radiation (about 70 percent had 3D conformal radiation therapy) after surgery.

Here is what the randomized NSABP B-39/RTOG 0413 (NRG Oncology) trial showed (when comparing whole breast radiation therapy with RT just to the region where the tumor had been removed), with half of the women followed for more than 10 years:

	Whole breast RT	Partial breast RT
10 year in-breast control	**95.9%**	**95.2%**
Recurrence-free survival	6.6%	8.1%
Disease-free survival	same	
Overall survival	same	

Although the trial could not declare statistical equivalence in controlling in-breast tumor recurrence, there are subsets of patients for whom PBI may be appropriate. In addition, the differences in local control are statistically significant, but clinically the results are almost identical.

Partial breast irradiation may be done with external beam using a linear accelerator, or as brachytherapy (here the radiation is inserted by a device temporarily into the breast). In the NRG study, 800 of 2000 patients who got partial breast irradiation had brachytherapy-based partial breast radiation therapy. While we need longer-term follow-up and monitoring before we can regard partial breast irradiation as equivalent to a more traditional approach using whole breast radiation therapy, for appropriately selected patients it is an excellent approach.

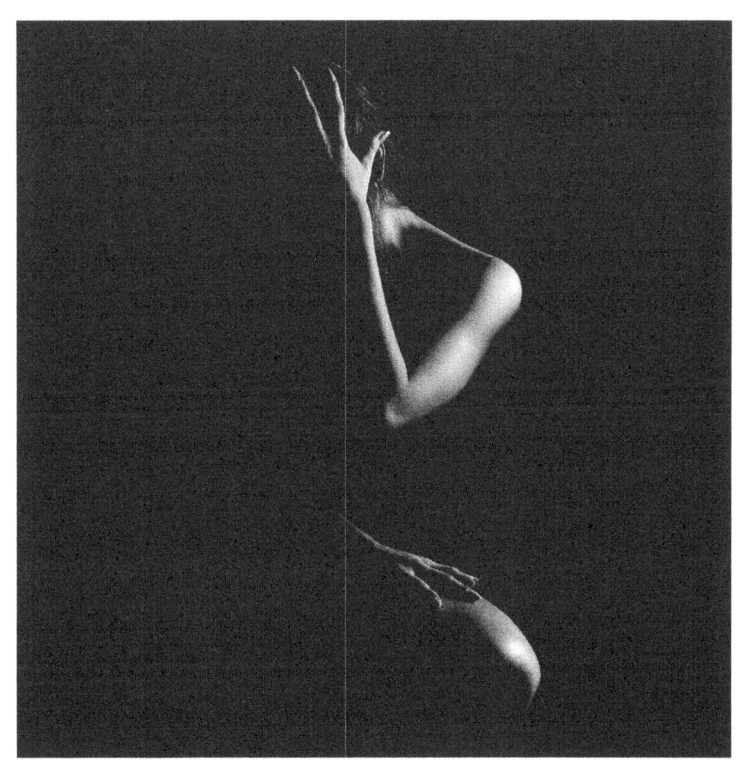

Management: Radiation after surgery

A challenge: Excess heart disease

Left breast or chest wall radiotherapy can deliver dose to the heart and coronary vessels, raising the risk of future cardiac events, including death. In an analysis of heart disease in a Nordic group of survivors of breast cancer, researchers found a significant excess risk associated with radiation therapy, a finding consistent with the risks seen in other radiotherapy-treated groups.

One potential solution: Respiratory gating

If radiation therapy hits the heart, it can potentially cause heart attack or even cardiovascular death. Today, we have innovative means to protect the heart. Respiratory gating software can be integrated into the radiation treatment plan. Your radiation oncologist can then define a physical window (like a baseball strike zone) and deliver radiation therapy only when the target is in this strike zone as you breath in and out. This technique can lead to the sparing of a greater amount of normal tissue such as the heart.

Example: Varian Real-time Position Management

This non-invasive, video-based approach allow clinicians to correlate target position in relation to your breathing cycle. Using an infrared tracking camera and a reflective marker, the sustem measures your respiratory patterns and displays them as a waveform. Your radiation oncologist then sets gating thresholds so that the radiation therapy beam turns off if your movement leaves you outside of preset limits.

Example: Elekta Versa HD system

Active Breathing Coordinator helps patients pause their breathing at a precisely indicated volume - a deep-inspiration breast-hold - which increases the distance between the tumor and critical structures, resulting in the ability to reduce doses to critical structures.

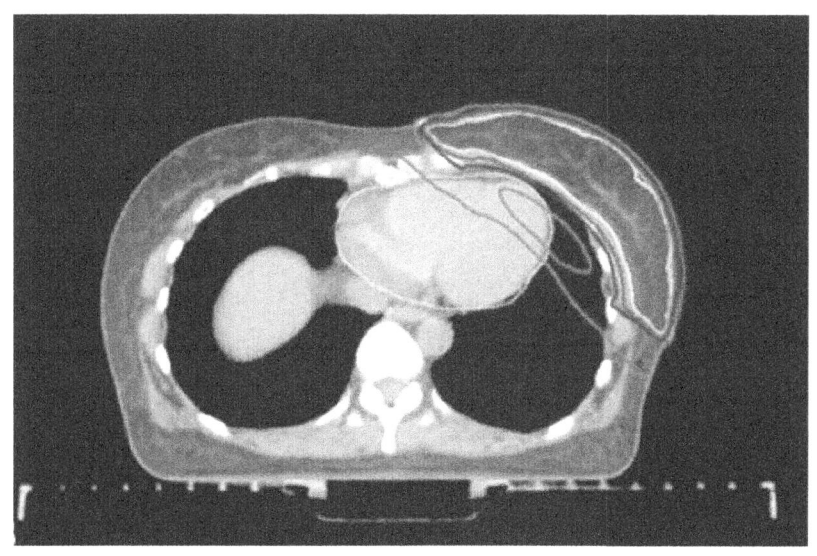

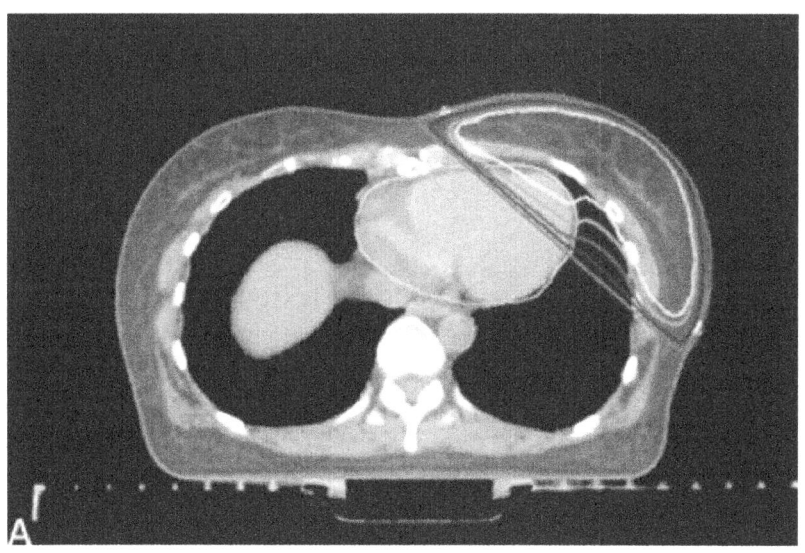

Short-term side effects

Whole breast radiation therapy may be associated with side effects, including breast skin fibrosis/scarring (4 percent), and decreased range of motion (1 percent). Mild generalized fatigue is common, often lasting for a month or two after completion of radiation therapy.

Longer-term side effects

• **Lymphedema:** Both surgery and radiation therapy can lead to early or delayed swelling of the breast, chest, or arm. Risks are highest among those who have a mastectomy with axillary node dissection followed by chest wall and axillary (underarm nodes) radiation therapy.

• **Nerve injury:** Uncommonly, RT can cause brachial plexopathy, damage to a nerve bundle at the top of your chest. This can cause weakness, or a tingling/burning sensation in the arm or hand. RT to the nodes around the collarbone may cause nerve injury in less than 1 percent of patients.

• **Lungs:** Radiation therapy to the breast region can result in lung inflammation (pneumonitis). Patients who have it may present with a persistent dry cough or shortness of breath. With today's techniques, pneumonitis is rare.

• **Heart:** Incidental radiation to the heart (as a part of treatment to the chest wall region for **left-sided cancers**) can result in a myriad of heart problems. These can include coronary artery disease, heart muscle injury, valve problems, and others. Technique matters greatly: Historic approaches often delivered relatively large doses to the heart or its vessels.

Once we recognized the radiation therapy side effects, we modified treatment techniques to substantially reduce heart irradiation. This is especially important for those who have received chemotherapy (or other drugs) that can damage the heart.

We have gotten better: In a study from the US Surveillance, Epidemiology, and End Results (SEER) database, the risk of death among those treated from 1973 to 1989 from ischemic heart disease was 13.1 versus 10.2 percent, when comparing left breast cancers to right ones. **For 1985 to 1989, the fifteen year death rates were not significantly different when comparing left and right side radiation therapy.** In our center, we use an innovative respiratory gating system, wherein the heart falls away from the target left chest wall, at which time the radiotherapy is delivered.

inspire

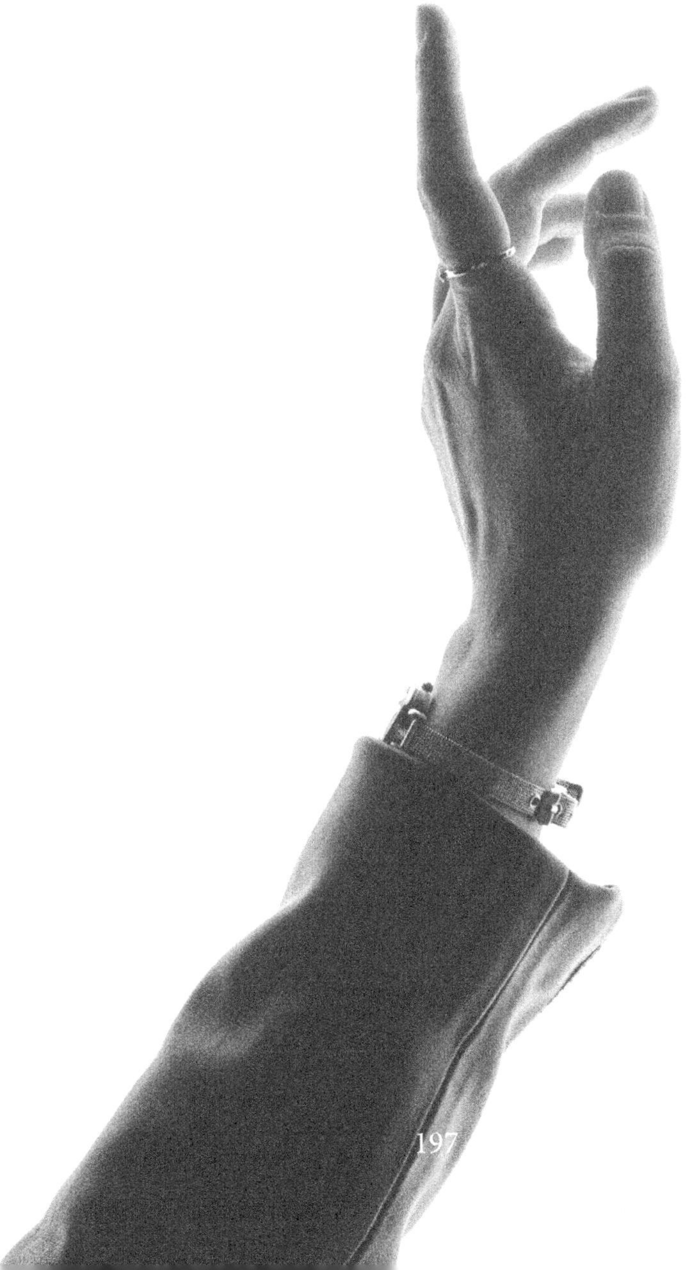

Management: Radiation therapy (RT) side effects

- **Musculoskeletal:** Breast and axillary surgery can cause reduced arm mobility. RT can worsen surgery-related pain and motor restriction in both the short- and long-term. Rib fractures from modern radiation therapy are uncommon, with a median time of about a year to its development.

- **Radiation therapy can uncommonly cause cancer,** including a 1 in 1000 risk of an aggressive angiosarcoma. The risk increases with dose, length of time after RT, and with younger age at the time of RT. We'll turn to other potential side effects of radiation therapy over the next couple of pages.

Leukemia

Rarely, radiation therapy can induce this blood cancer, or a condition known as myelodysplastic syndrome.

Lung cancer

The risk of lung cancer is higher among women who have had radiation therapy after a mastectomy as a part of treatment. The risk may not be increased for women who have had radiation therapy to the breast after a lumpectomy. The increased risk is first seen approximately ten years after radiation therapy, and can increase over time. The risk is higher for those who smoke cigarettes.

Sarcoma

Radiation therapy to the breast/chest wall region can increase your risk of a sarcoma of the blood vessels (angiosarcoma), bone (osteosarcoma), and other connective tissues in the radiation therapy volume. Fortunately, the risk if quite low.

Summary

Breast cancer treatment rarely causes cancer. The risk of a new primary non-breast cancer after breast cancer treatment is nicely illustrated by a review of 58,068 Dutch patients diagnosed with invasive breast cancer between 1989 and 2003. With a median follow-up of 5.4 years, here is what they discovered:

Radiation-induced cancer: Under 50 years old

Radiation therapy increases lung cancer risk 2.31-fold. Interestingly chemotherapy for this age group actually *decreased* second non-breast cancers (including colon and lung cancer) by a relative 22 percent.

Radiation-induced cancer: Over 50 years old

Radiation therapy increases the second non-breast cancer risk by a factor of 3.43.

We as caregivers should remain alert to the occurrence of second non-breast cancers. And you may reduce your risk with physical activity, a balanced diet, refraining from smoking, and optimizing your weight.

Recurrence

With appropriate management, the prognosis or patients with DCIS is excellent. An analysis of over 100,000 patients with DCIS enrolled in a national database in the USA found the 20 year disease-specific survival to approach 97%. The risk of same breast recurrence at 20 years was 5.9 percent, and the risk of other breast invasive disease was 6.2 percent. In this review, predictors of higher risk for death from breast cancer included young age at diagnosis (those under 35 had a 2.16-times increase in risk), high-grade (risk increased by 1.88-times), and black ethnicity (2.55-fold increase in risk).

Approximately one-half of all local recurrences are invasive, regardless of the initial treatment approach. Management hinges on the extent of disease, location, and prior surgical approach (mastectomy versus lumpectomy). **For patients with an invasive local recurrence after management for DCIS, consideration may be given to staging studies to check for distant spread of cancer.** There should also be a check on the recurrence disease for estrogen/progresterone receptor and HER2 statuses.

Original treatment	Management for local recurrence
Lumpectomy + RT*	Mastectomy
Lumpectomy with no RT*	Repeat lumpectomy + radiation therapy *or* mastectomy
Mastectomy	Excision of recurrence in mastectomy flap, then *consider* radiation therapy

* RT = Radiation therapy

Into the Future

Genomic testing

The Oncotype DX test examines the DCIS that has already been removed during your original surgery. The Oncotype DX DCIS test analyzes the activity of 12 genes and then estimates a woman's recurrence risk of DCIS (ductal carcinoma *in situ*) and/or the risk of a new invasive cancer developing in the same breast, as well as how likely she is to benefit from radiation therapy after DCIS surgery.

The DCIS Score is reported as a number between 0 and 100, is represented in two graphs. One graph shows the chances of any breast event (*either* DCIS or invasive breast cancer), while the other. A lower DCIS Score result means there is a lower chance that this will occur, and a higher score means that there is a higher chance that this will occur. The other graph represents the chances of the tumor coming back in the same breast as an *invasive* breast cancer. A lower score means there is a lower chance that this will occur, and a higher score means that there is a higher chance that this will occur.

The DCIS Score results can help guide personalized management decisions. Because everyone's DCIS is unique, a DCIS Score may help facilitate creating a treatment approach tailored to you. Here are the local recurrence rates in a study validating the OncoType DX test, at a median follow-up of 9.6 years:

- Low risk score: 13%
- Intermediate risk score: 28%
- High-risk score: 33%

Additional validation is needed before we can routinely use this test. Those who have an OncoType DX for DCIS should have a discussion balancing the recurrence reduction associated with radiation therapy with its risks.

MANAGEMENT

ENDOCRINE

Endocrine

"Anti-estrogen therapy

> **Action Point**
> Endocrine therapy (that targets estrogen that is feeding estrogen receptor positive DCIS) can reduce the risk of cancer events in the affected breast, while also halving the risk of breast cancer developing in the opposite (contralateral) breast. Endocrine therapy does not improve the odds of survival for those with ductal carcinoma *in situ*.

Background

Some DCIS cells use estrogen and/or progesterone ("female" hormones produced in the body) to fuel their own growth. When these hormones attach to proteins called hormone receptors, the cancer cells with these receptors grow. All breast cancers are checked to see if they are estrogen receptor-positive (ER +) or estrogen receptor-negative (ER -). The pathologist determines the receptor status by testing the tumor tissue removed during a biopsy or surgery. Most breast cancers are hormone receptor-positive. **"Hormone" (endocrine) therapies are known to have benefit for those with estrogen receptor-positive DCIS.**

How do they work?

"Anti-estrogen" (endocrine) therapies slow or stop the growth of hormone receptor-positive tumors by preventing the cancer cells from getting the hormones they need to grow. Some hormone therapies (for example, tamoxifen) attach to the receptor in the cancer cell, therefore blocking estrogen from attaching to the receptor. An alternative approach lowers estrogen levels in the body, depriving cancer cells of the estrogen they need to grow. The aromatase inhibitors are examples of this second approach, but are only used for women who no longer menstruate.

0.5

THAT'S THE RELATIVE RISK OF DEVELOPING A CANCER IN THE OPPOSITE BREAST (FOR THOSE WHO TAKE TAMOXIFEN FOR FIVE YEARS)*

* as compared with no tamoxifen

Naming

I prefer the terms endocrine therapy, or anti-estrogen treatment. Others use the somewhat confusing term "hormone therapy." The so-called hormone therapy used as a treatment for breast cancer is very different from that which is used as horonal replacement therapy for women struglling with symptoms related to menopause.

Because the endocrine therapy approach can hinge on your menopausal status, we should first define menopause:

> **menopause** [men'-uh-pawz]. noun.
> The National Comprehensive Cancer Network (www.nccn.org) considers women 50 and older to be post-menopausal if they have not had periods for 1 year or more (in the absence of tamoxifen, chemotherapy, or ovarian suppression) and the estradiol blood level is in the post-menopausal range. Women are also considered to be postmenopausal if there have been have no menstrual cycles while on tamoxifen and the estradiol blood levels are in the postmenopausal range.

There are several approaches to blocking hormones such as estrogen from driving the growth of an estrogen receptor-positive breast cancer:

- Selective estrogen receptor modulator (tamoxifen)
- Aromatase inhibitors, which block the conversion of androgens ("male" hormone) to estrogens (for example, aromatase inhibitors such as anastrazole (Arimidex), letrozole (Femara), and exemestane.
- Reduction (or destruction) or ovary function

Examples of aromatase inhibitors include anastrazole (brand name Arimidex); letrozole (Femara); and exemestane (Aromasin). These drugs are only for women in menopause, as they block the creation of estrogen in the body fat and adrenal glands, but do not block estrogen production from the ovaries. Some women discontinue an aromatase inhibitor within the first five years. It is considered reasonable to then switch to tamoxifen after at least two years of the aromatase inhibitor drug have been completed.

Aromatase inhibitor (AI) benefits

	Aromatase inhibitors versus tamoxifen
AI (5 years) versus tamoxifen (5 years)	From years 0 to 1, the AI dropped recurrence by 1/3 (relative risk 0.64); from years 2 to 4, the relative risk dropped by 1/5. After 5 years, there was no further impact on recurrence.
Tamoxifen (5 years) versus tamoxifen for 2-3 years, followed by AI (total 5 years of endocrine therapy)	From years 2 to 4, the AI-containing group had recurrence drop by nearly 1/2 (relative risk 0.56); After 5 years, there was no further impact on recurrence. There appeared to be fewer deaths from breast cancer associated with the switch to an aromatase inhibitor.
AI (5 years) versus tamoxifen (2-3 years) followed by an AI (total 5 years of endocrine therapy)	From years 0 to 1, the AI lowered recurrence rates (relative risk 0.74) compared to tamoxifen. From years 2 to 4, there were similar recurrence risks. Finally, the use of the AI alone led to a trend towards reduced breast cancer mortality, but it did not reach statistical significance (relative risk 0.89).

AIs and premenopausal women

Aromatase inhibitors (AIs) don't normally work in pre-menopausal women because their ovaries are still making estrogen, and the drugs don't block estrogen in the ovaries. However, some pre-menopausal women may take an aromatase inhibitor when combined with ovarian suppression (for example, drugs* that shut down the ovarian function), which shuts down the ovaries. Indeed, some findings suggest ovarian suppression plus an aromatase inhibitor may reduce breast cancer recurrence better than ovarian suppression plus tamoxifen (rates of freedom from breast cancer: 91 versus 87 percent at 68 months follow-up). This improvement is reflects reductions in local, regional, and contralateral breast events and in distant recurrence.

* examples include leuprolide (Lupron) and goserelin (Zoladex); alternatively, the ovaries may be surgically removed.

DCIS: Management with endocrine therapy

Tamoxifen (for 5 years)

Tamoxifen is an "anti-estrogen" pill. The NSABP B-24 randomized trial showed tamoxifen can reduce the probability of future events in the breast treated for DCIS, as well as in the opposite (contralateral) breast among women with DCIS who undergo lumpectomy followed by radiation therapy. There are clear benefits if the DCIS is estrogen receptor-positive (ER +).

Evidence for benefit

The NSABP B-24 trial was randomized clinical trial that randomized women with DCIS to either lumpectomy and radiation versus the same treatment followed by the anti-estrogen pill tamoxifen (taken for 5 years). The study showed the following at 17 year follow-up:

- Tamoxifen lowered the risk of a future invasive or non-invasive cancer in *either* breast. The risk of *invasive* cancer dropped by 6 per 1000 to 19 per 1000, or about one-third (relative risk 0.68);

- Tamoxifen benefit appeared limited to women with estrogen receptor positive DCIS.

A United Kingdom Coordinating Committee on Cancer Research study found:

- Tamoxifen did *not* lower the risk of invasive cancer in the same breast, but did lower the risk of invasive cancer in the opposite breast. The researchers did not provide absolute reduction numbers.

- Tamoxifen lowered the risk of DCIS recurrence in the same breast.

- Tamoxifen *did not* lower the risk of DCIS in the opposite breast.

Meta-analysis (Putting the Studies Together)

- Tamoxifen lowers the risk of a future ipsilateral (same) invasive breast cancer by about one-fifth (relative risk 0.79).
- Tamoxifen lowers the risk of a future contralateral (other breast) event risk by nearly half (relative risk 0.57).

Aromatase inhibitor (AI) pills trump tamoxifen

Treatment of *postmenopausal* women with DCIS with the aromatase inhibitor anastrozole resulted in higher breast cancer–free survival rates compared with standard treatment with tamoxifen. The NSABP B-35/SWOG-35 study randomized 3,104 postmenopausal women with hormone receptor–positive DCIS to either daily 20 mg tamoxifen or 1 mg anastrozole for 5 years. All patients had a lumpectomy and radiation therapy prior to starting their 5-year regimen of "anti-estrogen" pills. Here are the results with a median follow-up of 8.6 years:

- Patients on anastrozole were about a quarter less likely to recur, at least compared to their counterparts who took tamoxifen.
- Anastrozole appeared to reduce the diagnosis of a second primary breast cancer in the opposite breast, but this trend was not quite statistically significant.

Tamoxifen and the aromatase inhibitor pill anastrazole can reduce the future event probability in either breast. The availability of both drugs means we have choices for postmenopausal women, so we can now better customize therapy for the individual. Premenopausal women have tamoxifen as a potential treatment tool, particularly if their DCIS is estrogen receptor-positive (ER +).

Systemic therapy

For patients who have had appropriate management of the breast (in which the cancer recurred), consideration may be given adding systemic therapy to surgery. This is especially true if the recurrence is invasive (infiltrating). For some, this may mean anti-estrogen approaches such as tamoxifen or an aromatase inhibitor pill (for example, if the invasive cancer is estrogen receptor-positive). Selected patients with higher risk disease may receive chemotherapy, and those whose invasive recurrence is positive for HER2 (human epidermal growth factor receptor-2) should receive a HER2-directed drug such as trastazumab (Herceptin).

The decision to incorporate ovarian suppression for those at high-risk is challenging as there can be significant side effects associated with this approach. There does not appear to be a benefit for those *not* at higher risk of recurrence.

Side effects: Tamoxifen

A meta-analysis (anlysis of a collection of studies) from the 2011 Early Breast Cancer Trialists' Collaborative Group compared tamoxifen for five years versus no endocrine therapy. Here are some (but not all) of the major side effects found to be associated with tamoxifen:

- Deep venous thrombosis (blood clots, for example in your calf)
- Uterus cancer (limited to women over 55 years of age)
- Hot flashes
- Vaginal discharge
- Sexual dysfunction
- Menstrual irregularities
- Stroke (not statistically significant)

Hot flashes

Hot flashes are among the most common and troublesome toxicities of tamoxifen. They are thought due to a central nervous system anti-estrogen effect resulting in dysfunction of your body heat regulation system. Up to 80 percent of women on tamoxifen get hot flashes; for 30 percent they are severe.

There is variability among individuals in hot flash risk associated with tamoxifen. For example, premenopausal women are more likely to get them, compared to postmenopausal women. Genetics may play a role, too. In addition, some anti-depressant drugs known as SSRIs can decrease the conversion of tamoxifen to its most active byproduct (endoxiphen), influencing your chances of getting hot flashes. Examples include paroxetine and fluoxetine.

Blood clots

Tamoxifen can increase the risk of so-called thromboembolic disease, including pulmonary embolism (clots in the lung) and stroke. This elevated risk continues as long as you are on the drug. There may be additional risk when tamoxifen is added to chemotherapy, and he risk appears to rise if the tamoxifen is extended from 5 to 10 years.

Side effects: Tamoxifen (continued)

 Risk factors for developing clots in your veins also include prior surgery, fracture, and immobilization. Your doctor may counsel you to discontinue the tamoxifen for several days prior to prolonged immobilization from planned surgery or travel.

An analysis of trials of tamoxifen from the Early Breast Cancer Trialists Collaborative Group demonstrated a non-significant excess of stroke deaths (3 extra per 1000 women during the first 15 years), but this risk was exactly balanced by a reduction in heart-related deaths (3 fewer per 1000 women).

Endometrial (uterus) cancer

Tamoxifen can raise the risk of both the common type of uterus cancer and a less common one known as uterine sarcoma. In the Early Breast Cancer Trialists Collaborative Group overview analysis of 20 trials, researchers found tamoxifen to be associated with a 2.4-fold increased risk of uterus cancer, but there was no increase in deathlinked to this increase in risk. The rate in the Breast Cancer Prevention Trial was 2.3 per 1,000 women per year, compared to 0.9 for the placebo group.

With long-term follow-up, we now know that tamoxifen results in a very small increase in the incidence of an uncommon cancer of the uterus: Uterine sarcoma (carcinosarcoma or mixed Mullerian tummors) risk increases.The absolute risk of MMMT results in an additional 1.4 cases per 10,000 women per year.

Other tumors

While most individual clinical trials (including the largest one, the P-1 trial) looking at tamoxifen did *not* show an increases in non-uterine cancer, a meta-analysis of 16 randomized trials comparing tamoxifen with a placebo suggested a 1.3-fold increase in **gastrointestinal cancers.** We have some hints that tamoxifen may *lower* your risk of **ovarian cancer.** Still, we do not have high-level evidence to assert this with confidence.

Childbearing

Women of childbearing potential whould use an effective menas of contraception. Indeed, tamoxifen can induce ovulation. After stopping, check with your physician to see if you should be off the drug a minimum of a few months to ensure the drug has cleared your system.

Side effects: Tamoxifen (continued)

Coronary heart disease

Among postmenopausal women, tamoxifen may not be associated with either a beneficial or adverse cardiovascular effect. Still, the data are mixed. While tamoxifen can improve your lipid profile, it has not consistently been linked to a beneficial heart effect.

Eye problems

Tamoxifen has been found in some (but not all) studies to be linked to an increased risk of cataracts. The drug has been linked to dry eye, irritation, and retinal deposits that may cause macular edema. However, these side effects are uncommon. Your first line of defense? A baseline eye exam.

Other

Tamoxifen has been associated with vaginal discharge, menstrual irregularities, sexual dysfunction, and other problems.

Childbearing age

Women of childbearing potential should use effective contraception while on tamoxifen, as the drug can induce ovulation and also raise the risk of congenital abnormalities. After stopping tamoxifen, check with your physician to see if you should be off the drug for a minimum of a few months (before attempting to conceive a child) to ensure the drug has cleared out.

Side effects: Aromatase inhibitors (AIs)

- Musculoskeletal problems (bone pain, joint stiffness/achiness): Severe in about 1/3 patients, although the difference between placebo (inactive "fake" pill) versus aromatase inhibitors in randomized trials appears to be about 5 to 8 percent. Still, 10 to 20% will quit the AI because of these symptoms.
- Sexual dysfunction, pain, or dissatisfaction
- Reduced vaginal lubrication; reduced sexual interest
- Cognitive problems (forgetfulness, for example)
- Fatigue

Musculoskeletal (muscle/bone) syndrome

Aromatase inhibitors can be associated with joint pain or stiffness, and/or muscle or bone pain. For about a third of patients this symptom can be severe; on the other hand if we look at the difference between aromatase inhibitor and placebo (inert), there is a 5 to 8 percent difference. The bottom line? Musculoskeletal symptoms lead 10 to 20 percent of patients to stop the medicine.

The good news? There appears to be a dose-response relationship between exercise and symptom severity, at least according to the Hormones and Physical Exercise (HOPE) trial. The exercise regimen consisted of twice-weekly supervised resistance and strength training plus moderate aerobic exercise for 150 minutes per week. Other patients use non-steroidal anti-inflammatory drugs, but they have their own potential risks. Sometimes a switch to a different aromatase inhibitor can be beneficial. Some believe the antidepressant and nerve pain medication doxetine (Cymbalta) may provide some relief for patients for whom a switch to a differnt AI doesn't help. Finally, vitamin D might help. One study used vitamin D2, 50,000 IU capsule per week, and found it to be helpful. Still, such high-doses of vitamin D require close monitoring of blood levels.

Sexual dysfunction

Use of an aromatase inhibitor can result in vaginal symptoms and sexual dysfunction. Some patients describe reduced sexual interest, while others report diminished vaginal lubrication and/or pain with sex. Others mention orgasmic dysfunction and general dissatisfaction with their sex life.

Other side effects

Some women describe cognitive challenges associated with the use of an aromatase inhibitor. In fact, predictors of discontinuation of the drug by one year included:

- Fatigue
- Forgetfulness
- Poor sleep

Compared to tamoxifen, aromatase inhibitor use is linked with a *higher* risk of bone loss (osteoporosis), bone fractures, cardiovascular problems, and elevated cholesterol levels. On the positive side, aromatase inhibitor use can lead to a *lower* risk of venous thrombous (blood clots in your veins) and endometrial (uterus) cancer, at least as cmopared with tamoxifen.

Preferred aromatase inhibitor (AI)

The aromatase inhibitors drugs, compared with one another, seem to have equivalent effectiveness when used in the adjuvant setting (following surgery with curative intent).

Timing of aromatase inhibitor (AI)

No chemotherapy, no radiation therapy

If you have hormone receptor positive breast cancer, and are not scheduled to have chemotherapy or radiation therapy, most patients begin the AI about four to six weeks following surgery.

Chemotherapy

For patients getting chemotherapy, it is generally recommended to sequence the chemotherapy before the endocrine therapy, although a meta-analysis from the Early Breast Cancer Trialists' Collaborative Group that compared concurrent with sequential treatment found similar drops in the risk for recurrence.

Radiation therapy

For women receiving radiotherapy after surgery, some clinicians have you start the aromatase inhibitor during radiation, while others wait until radiation therapy is complete. This author is unaware of data showing a difference in survival based on the timing of AI initiation relative to radiation therapy.

HER-2 positive

In the original clinical trials showing tremendous value for the addition of trastazumab (Herceptin) to chemotherapy for HER-2 overexpressing breast cancer, endocrine therapy was initiated (for hormone receptor positive cancers) once the chemotherapy portion of treatment was complete.

Non-compliance

One large study suggests that non-compliance with either tamoxifen or an aromatase inhibitor may increase your risk of death overall, although there appeared to be no influence on breast cancer-specific mortality. We join the National Comprehensive Cancer Network (NCCN) in encouraging compliance with recommended endocrine therapy, if you opt to do it.

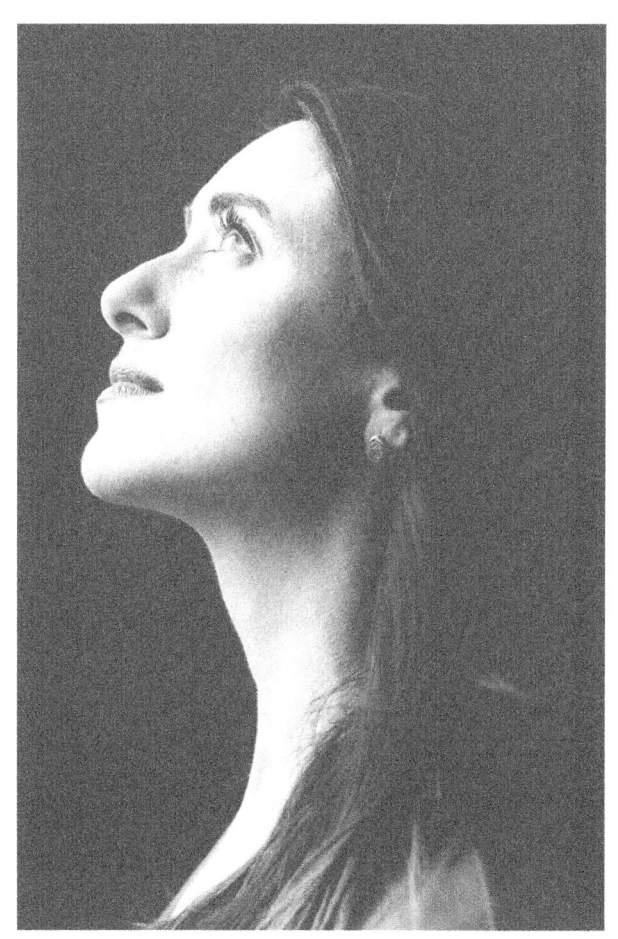

MANAGEMENT
IN-BREAST RELAPSE

Recurrence

With appropriate management, the prognosis or patients with DCIS is excellent. An analysis of over 100,000 patients with DCIS enrolled in a national database in the USA found the 20 year disease-specific survival to approach 97%. The risk of same breast recurrence at 20 years was 5.9 percent, and the risk of other breast invasive disease was 6.2 percent. In this review, predictors of higher risk for death from breast cancer included young age at diagnosis (those under 35 had a 2.16-times increase in risk), high-grade (risk increased by 1.88-times), and black ethnicity (2.55-fold increase in risk).

Approximately one-half of all local recurrences are invasive, regardless of the initial treatment approach. Management hinges on the extent of disease, location, and prior surgical approach (mastectomy versus lumpectomy). **For patients with an invasive local recurrence after management for DCIS, consideration may be given to staging studies to check for distant spread of cancer.** There should also be a check on the recurrence disease for estrogen/progresterone receptor and HER2 statuses.

Original treatment	Management for local recurrence
Lumpectomy + RT*	Mastectomy
Lumpectomy with no RT*	Repeat lumpectomy + radiation therapy *or* mastectomy
Mastectomy	Excision of recurrence in mastectomy flap, then *consider* radiation therapy

* RT = Radiation therapy

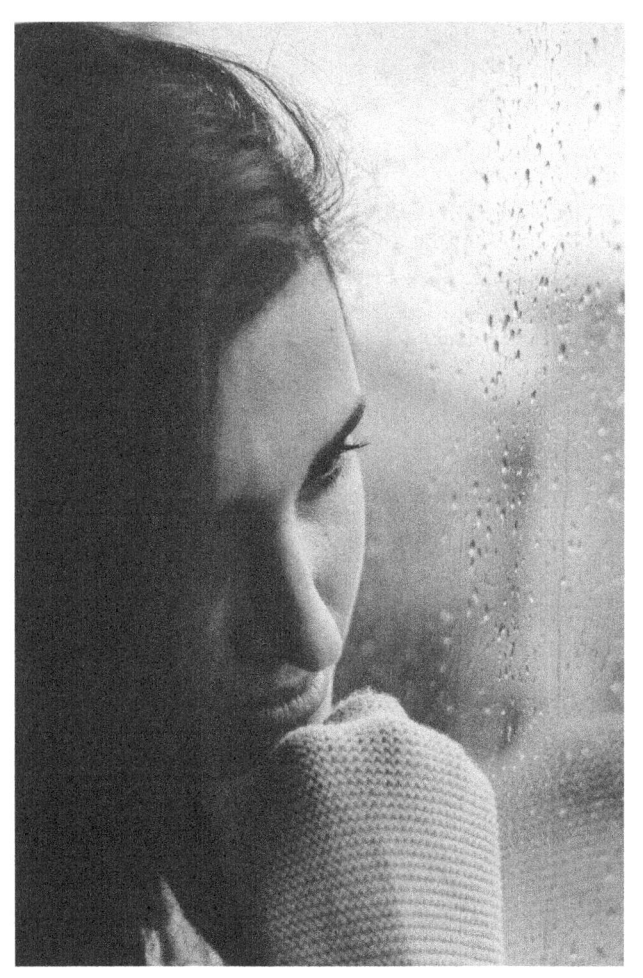

Metastases: Uncommon

Distant spread of cancer (3% of DCIS)

> metastasis [muh-TAS-tuh-sis]: the development of secondary cancer growths at a distance from a primary site of cancer.

As the risk of distant spread of DCIS is low, I will only touch on some basics. Distant spread of cancer is sometimes referred to as advanced, metastatic or stage IV (4) breast cancer. What all of these mean is that cancer has spread from the orignial site in the breast to more distant parts of the body. The most common sites of spread include the bones, liver, and lung. The cancer can also spread to the brain or other body parts, however. In addition, metastatic cancer can affect one or more locations simultaneously. Spread to regional regions such as the axillary (underarm) nodes, paraclavicular (above or below the collarbone) nodes, or internal mammary nodes (next to the breastbone or sternum) may occur, but these are regional (and not distant) sites of spread.

How does distant spread occcur?

Metastatic breast cancer develops when cells from the original cancer in the breast travel to distant parts of the body through the blood or lymphatic system. This new cancer is still known as breast cancer, even though it is in a different body part. Sometimes the cancer is present in distant sites at diagnosis, either macroscopically (we know about the metastases) or microscopically (our tests cannot show the distant spread, but it is present in small amounts). Alternatively, some cancer cells may survive treatment for what is initially non-metastatic cancer.

We have long believed that cancer metastasizes (spreads) when a single cancer cell escapes from the original tumor, travels through the bloodstream and sets up shop in distant organs. However, a growing body of evidence suggests that these bad actors don't travel alone; instead **cancer cells migrate through the body in cellular clusters, like gangs.** Roaming tumor clumps are led by a gang member that's fueled by a type of cellular kryptonite: a highly expressed protein called keratin 14. Understanding the molecular basis of collective dissemination may enable novel prognostics and therapies to improve patient outcomes.

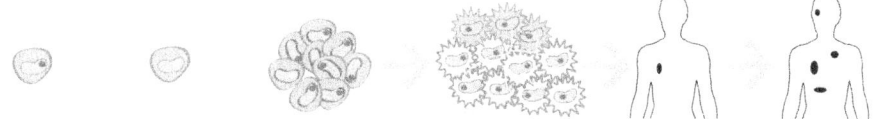

RESTORE

Breast reconstruction

Restoration

Breast reconstruction: Basics

You may have had (or be about to have) a removal of your breast(s). Some will have a mastectomy as a part of treatment, while others do it vecause they are at very high risk of developing breast cancer in the future. Breast reconstruction, if performed, often takes place during the mastectomy procedure. Some patients elect delayed reconstruction, to be performed months or even years after the breast removal. Less commonly, patients desire reconstruction after a lumpectomy.

Losing a breast can be traumatic. Some patients feel sad, anxious, or mournful. Now, you may be offered the opportunity to reconstruct your breast. Some women simply choose not to reconstruct. So how do you decide? You may wish to consider:

- How important is your breast to you?
- Would you be comfortable with a prosthesis, a breast form that you take on and off?
- Will reconstruction help you to feel more whole?
- Are you comfortable with additional surgery and the potential associated complications?

Please note that even if you choose reconstruction, it doesn't restore sensation to the breast or the nipple. Now, if you decide to proceed with breast reconstruction, there are two majoy categories:

- implant-based reconstruction (uses a saline, or salt water versus a silicone implant to create a breast shape;
- autologous (flap) reconstruction (uses tissue taken from another area of your body to create a breast form).

On occasion, a surgeon may combine the two approaches.

Reconstruction: Implants

Reconstruction using prosthetic devices ay be performed in eith one or two stages. For one-stage reconstruction, a permanent implant is inserted at the time of your mastectomy. With two-stage reconstruction, a tissue expander is placed at the same time as your breast removal, and gradually filled until you get to your desired size. The tissue expander is replaced by a permanent implant at a later date.

Reconstruction: Autologous

Here, you use your own tissues to create a new breast. Donor sites may be from the abdomen, back, inner thigh, or buttocks.

Reconstruction: Following oncoplastic surgery

Oncoplastic surgery involves the creation of a wider resection of the breast caner (as compared with traditional breast-conserving surgery), followed by immediate or delayed (but before radiation therapy) reconstruction of the breast deformity. Basically, there is tissue rearrangement as a means of restouring a more natural breast contour. Such surgery may allow for better margins than a traditional lumpectomy, decreasing the need for mastectomy (particularly for those with a larger breast cancer to breast size ratio).

Reconstruction: The nipple

After breast reconstruction, if the nipple has been removed as a part of your cancer operation, you may desure a nipple-areolar reconstruction. This is often done during the second stage of breast reconstruction. One of several techniques may be used. A tattooing procedure for the areola (colored area around the nipple) may be added to opimize the cosmetic outcome. Some patients will choose the creation of a 3-dimensional tattoo as an alternative to surgical reconstruction of the nipple.

Trouble? Tobacco, diabetes, obesity, COPD and more

Tobacco users have a significantly higher risk of surgical complications, especially with reconstruction using their own tissues. Obesity, insulin-dependent diabetes, chronic obstructive pulmonary disease, connective tissue disorders, and thrombophilia (an abnormality of blood coagulation that increases the risk of blood clots in blood vessels) can raise risk, too.

Restoration

Breast reconstruction: Timing

Breast reconstruction can be accomplished at the same time as a mastectomy (immediate) versus at a subsequent operation (delayed). Let's look first at the timing of reconstruction:

- *Immediate*

Years ago, delayed reconstruction was prederred, but there has been an evolution over time: Today, we know that immediate reconstruction can be associated with with significant psychological benefits. In addition, the surgery process is streamlined, as the breast removal and reconstruction can be done at one setting. Normal breast landmarks, including the junction of the breast and chest (inframammary fold) are preserved with immediate breast reconstruction.

Of course, there are potential downsides too. Immediate reconstruction prolongs the surgery time, adding an hour or more for implant-based reconstruction and even more for reconstructions using your own tissue. Some patients will have breakdown (necrosis) of the mastectomy skin flaps, negatively affecting the cosmetic outcome. Finally, those with large cancers, direct invasion of the skin or chest wall, or nodal involvement, or concerning margins (cancer-free zone around the removed breast) have a strong recommendation for radiation therapy (RT). RT can negatively impact your breast reconstruction.

- *Delayed*

Delayed reconstruction may be recommended if you have suboptimal blood flow to the skin flaps after mastectomy. Some patients who need radiation therapy, have significant other illnesses, or suboptimal social habits (obesity; poorly-controlled diabetes, tobacco usage) may need to delay reconstruction. Those with the locally advanced form of breast cancer known as inflammatory breast cancer should delay reconstruction, too.

Delayed reconstruction allows for assurance of clear margins prior to restoration. It can reduce the chances of having inadequate blood flow to the mastectomy skin flaps. Disadvantages include the need for surgery at a later date, often a less good cosmetic outcome (compared with immediate reconstruction), and limitations on reconstruction options after radiotherapy.

The optimal timing of reconstruction, relative to radiation therapy, remains controversial. Some advocate getting a quick look at a removed sentinel node at the time of surgery, and delaying reconstruction if the node is involved. An alternative for those getting implant-based reconstruction is to place a tissue expander at the time of the breast removal, preserving the shape of the breast envelope. After the final pathology report comes out several days to about a week later, those who don't need radiation therapy may procced to early completion of their reconstruction process; those that need RT may delay the final reconstruction. Please know, that your radiation oncologist may (or may not) request a temporary deflation of one or both tissue expanders to optimize radiation therapy targeting.

Implants associated with small risk of lymphoma

A study from 2018 found that one in 6,920 women with breast implants will develop an aggressive form of cancer known as anaplastic large-cell lymphoma (ALCL) in the breast before they reach age 75.

ALCL is a type of non-Hodgkin's lymphoma that can affect the skin, lymph nodes, or organs throughout the body. In the recent study, researchers examined the nationwide Dutch pathology registry to identify all cases of breast-ALCL in the country from 1990 to 2016. Among the 43 cases found, 32 were in women with breast implants. So-called macrotextured implants were found in 23 of 28 patients (for whom the implant type was known) with lymphoma; microtextured implants were found in the remaining five patients. **No smooth or polyurethane covered implants were seen in breast-ALCL patients.**

Restoration

Breast reconstruction: Impact of radiation

A minority of patients who have a mastectomy will need radiation therapy (RT), based on involvement of the nodes with cancer, concerning margins, or locally advanced disease. Radiation therapy can be problematic, as it increases the chance of complications associated with reconstruction.

- *Radiation therapy (RT) and implant complications*

Radiation therapy complications are highest among women who have expander/implant reconstruction, whether RT is given before or after the surgery. Complications may include scar formation at the impant/tissue interface, contracture of the capsule, or problems with healing od the skin. Some patients will experience implant rupture, have the implant rupture through the skin, or become badly positioned.

> In a study from Utah (USA), radiation therapy did *not* affect patient satisfaction. Still, radiation therapy led to a higher rate of breast implant removal. The **implant removal rates for non-radiation and radiation therapy patients were 4% and 22%,** respectively.

Implants placed in front of (instead of behind) the chest wall muscle may have a lower complication rate, but this is an evolving area.

- *Radiation therapy (RT) and autologous (flap) tissue complications*

Radiation therapy can result in flap shrinkage, necrosis (tissue death), flap shrinkage, or scarring. Still, flap-based reconstructions generally tolerate radiation therapy better than do implant-based ones. The incidence of late complications may be lower when flap-based reconstruction is done after (instead of prior to) radiation therapy. Stillcomplications are not uncommon: One retrospective study found a complication rate of 32 percent for those who had radiation therapy first, compared to 44 percent for those who had breasy reconstruction first.

Breast reconstruction: After

Walk

Your surgeon will likely ask you to begin walking soon after the operation. This can reduce the risk of your forming clots, a condition known as deep vein thrombosus (DVTs), and can improve your lung function as well.

Drains

Following an implant-based reconstruction, a drain is usually placed in the implant space, and will remain there for several days. By day 2 or 3 after surgery, most patients are allowed to shower. When a tissue expander is used, expansion in the office or clinic is typically done at one- or two-week intervals until complete. For a reconstruction using your own tissues, the duration of the drain is variable. Many patients are in the hospital for three to four days, and often can shower on post-operative days 2 or 3.

Discomfort

Many experience pain at the site of the incision and may experience spasms of local muscles. Perhaps not surprisingly, you will likely have to avoid strenuous activities for up to about six weeks after the surgery. As physicians, we are working hard to reduce the use of narcotic medications for pain. Enhanced recovery after surgery (ERAS) protocols include preoperative counseling, optimization of nutrition, standardized analgesic and anesthetic regimens and early mobilization. Ask your surgeon about what you can do to reduce your probability of having long-term problems with narcotics.

Don't forget to: 1) make the narcotic pain medications in your home inaccessible to others; 2) watch for constipation; 3) not operate heavy machinery (including automobiles); and 4) get the narcotics out of your home as soon as reasonable (for example, select pharmacies have boxes for trashing them).

Surveillance after breast reconstruction

Mastectomy is not a guarantee that there will not be a local recurrence. In that context, follow-up is important. The vast majority of local and regional recurrences are palpable; they can be felt. Thus, physical exam is central to the detection of recurrent breast cancer. Most feel that mammograms after reconstruction (following breast removal) are not necessary.

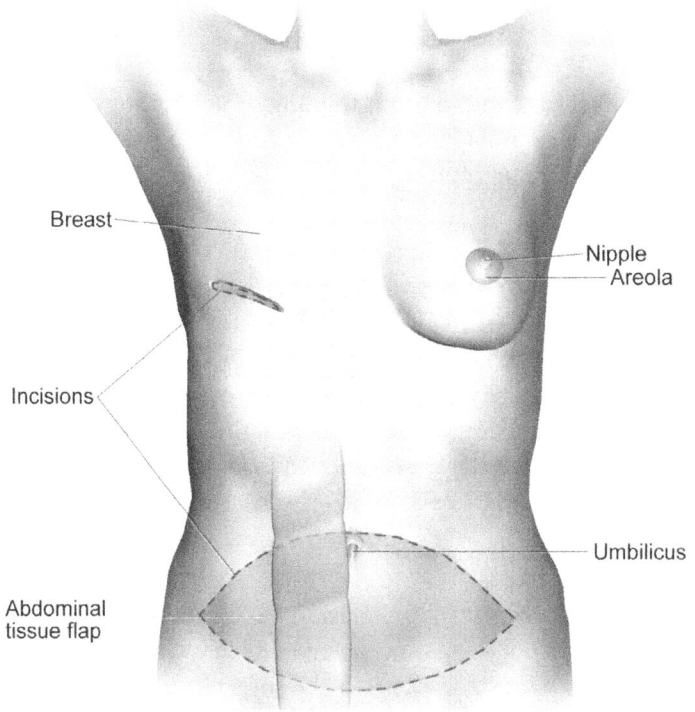

TRAM (transverse rectus abdominis) is a muscle in your lower abdomen between your waist and your pubic bone. A flap of this skin, fat, and all or part of the underlying rectus abdominus ("6-pack") muscle are used to reconstruct the breast in a TRAM flap procedure.

A DIEP flap is similar to a muscle-sparing free TRAM flap, except that no muscle is used to rebuild the breast. (A muscle-sparing free TRAM flap uses a small amount of muscle.) A DIEP flap is considered a muscle-sparing type of flap. DIEP stands for the deep inferior epigastric perforator artery, which runs through the abdomen.

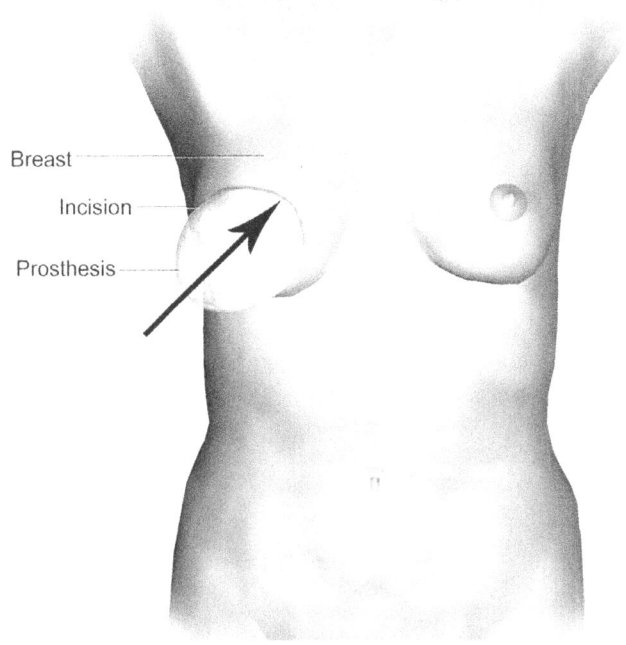

Implant-based reconstruction typically requires less extensive surgery than flap reconstruction, as it only involves the chest area and not tissue donor sites. Still, you may need additional surgery in the future, as implants can wear out (often within 10 to 20 years) or develp other issues (including scar tissue forming around the implant).

Implants may be filled with saline (salt water), silicone gel, or a combination of both. The implant itself is often placed behind the chest muscle. The device itself may be round or tear-shaped, and the surface may be smooth or have a slightly rough texture.

Restoration

Summary

Types

- Devices-based reconstruction
Tissue expanders; salt water-filled implants; silicone-filled implants

- Oncoplastic reconstruction
Volume displacement or replacement techniques)

- Autologous reconstruction
Involves the transfer of a flap of tissue from a donor site (for example, the abdomen or belly) to the front chest wall.

The choice of reconstruction depends on body shape, other medical problems (diabetes; smoking; obesity), the size and shape of the other breast, prior surgical procedures, the quality of the chest skin, and patient preference.

Timing
Breast reconstruction if often performed immediately after the breast removal; it may be done during the same operating room time. Immediate reconstruction allows for reduced costs, often better cosmetic outcomes, psycological benefits, and more streamlined care. Immediate reconstruction may be especially appealing for thoe who are haing a prophylactic (preventative or risk-reducing) breast removal, or a mastectomy for ductal carcinoma in sity or for invasive breast cancers that are 5 centimeters or less and are not known to be assoicated with spread ti regional lymph nodes.

For those who likely need radiation therapy after a mastecomt, delayed or so-called delayed-immediate reconstruction may be considered. Many surgeons don't like to irradiate a flap reconstruction, as there can be long-term complications. Still, autologous (your own tissues) reconstruction is often preferred (as compared to an implant) following radiation therapy, since there are fewer complications following the radiation therapy.

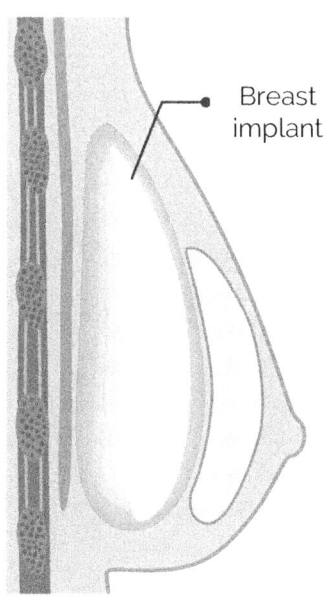

Subglandular insertion

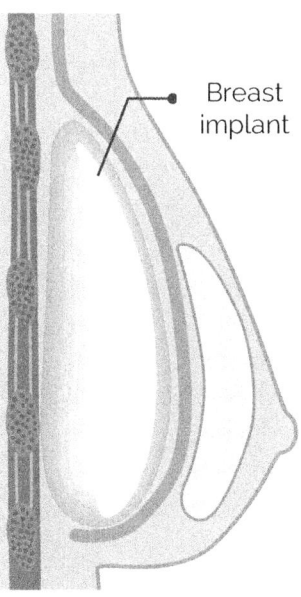

Submuscular insertion

SPECIAL

Pregnancy;
Paget's; Young

Pregnancy

Breast cancer during pregnancy

Breast cancer occurring with pregnancy is infrequent: A California study showed 1.3 breast cancers diagnosed per 10,000 live births. Alas, many such cancers are associated with spread to regional nodes, and often present with a larger cancer in the breast, more aggressive cancer cell characteristics, and are more likely to overexpress HER2 or be estrogen- and progesterone receptor negative.

Initial evaluation

The natural tenderness and engorgement of the breasts of pregnant and lactating women may make detection of early diagnosis of breast cancer challenging. Often, pregnancy-related cancers are detected at a later stage than in a non-pregnant, age-matched population.

Physical exam and imaging come first. Mammograms may be done (with protective shielding, there appears to be little risk of radiation exsposure to the fetus *after* the first trimester; still mammograms are used selectively). Because at least 25% of mammograms in pregnancy may be negative in the presence of cancer, a biopsy is essential for the diagnosis of any palpable mass.

Ultrasound An ultrasound of the breasts and regional lymph nodes allows for an assessment of the extent of disease.

Biopsy

While fine needle aspiration biopsies may be done, a core needle biopsy is preferred and allows for an assessment of the status of estrogen- and progesterone receptors (ER, PR), as well as HER2. Breast cancer pathology is similar in age-matched pregnant and nonpregnant women. However, elevated estrogen levels associated with pregnancy may lead to a higher incidence of ER detection with a test called immunohistochemistry, as to radiolabeled ligand-binding testing. Ask your doctor how your cancer was checked for estrogen receptors, as the radiolabeled ligand-binding test has a higher chance of finding estrogen receptors, important for prognosis and management.

Management

Assessment of the pregnancy should include a **maternal fetal medicine consultation** and review of current maternal risks such as hypertension, diabetes, and complications with prior pregnancies. You should have an assessment of fetal growth and development and fetal age with an ultrasound exam. Estimation of the date of the delivery can help with systemic chemotherapy planning, if this treatment is indicated. Maternal fetal medicine consultation should include counseling regarding maintaining or terminating pregnancy, although most women can maintain their pregnancy, in spite of the need for DCIS surgery.

In general, we manage early breast cancer in the same way as we do non-pregnant women. Of course, there can be some modifications in order to provide protection to the fetus. Breast cancer surgery appears to be safe during pregnancy. Although the anesthesia used during surgery can cross the placenta to the fetus, it fortunately doesn't appear to cause birth defects or serious pregnancy problems.

Surgery options for early breast cancer may include mastectomy versus breast conserving surgery and radiation. We cannot give **radiation therapy** to a pregnant woman, but if she is towards the end of her pregnancy (before radiation therapy would be given), breast conservation followed by delivery of the baby, in turn by radiation therapy may be an exellent option for select individuals.

Pregnancy after breast cancer treatment: Appears safe

While we do not have high level evidence, the available clinical literature suggest that women who have a pregnancy after having been managed for breast cancer do not compromise their own survival chances. In addition, there appear to be no harmful effects on the fetus. Still, given the recurrence risk is highest in the first couple of years after a breast cancer diagnosis, many prefer to wait for a period of time (for example, 2 years) before attempting to conceive.

No damaging effects on the fetus from maternal breast cancer have been demonstrated, and there are no reported cases of maternal-fetal transfer of breast cancer cells.

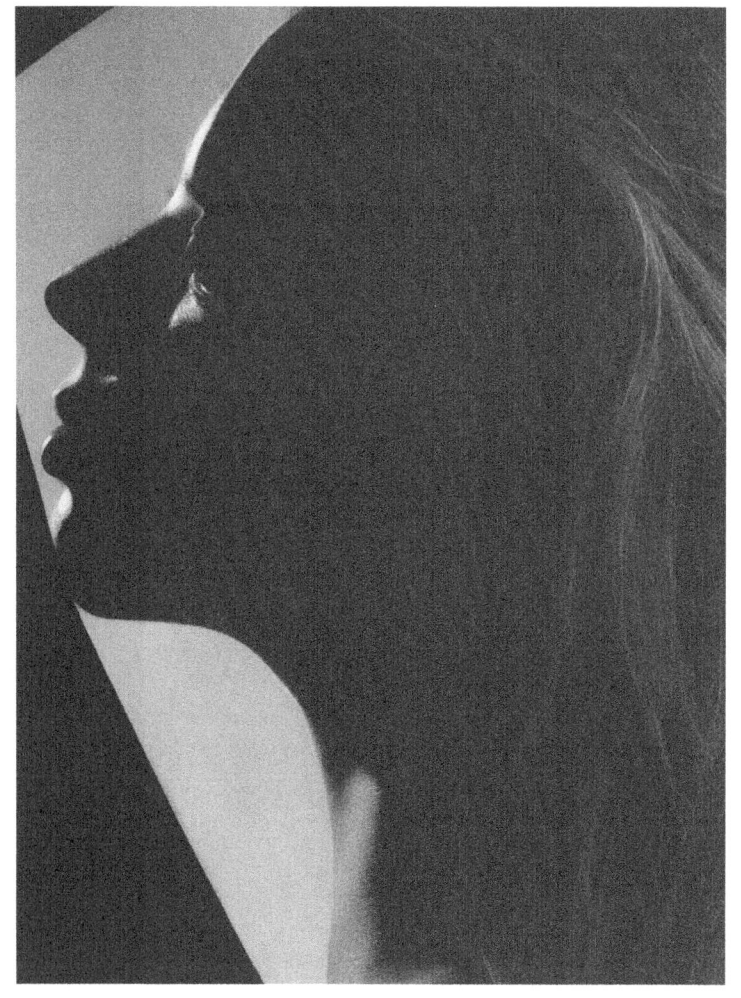

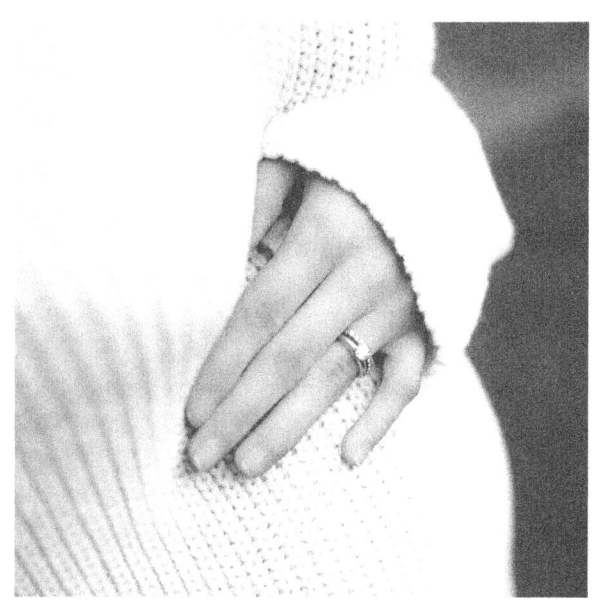

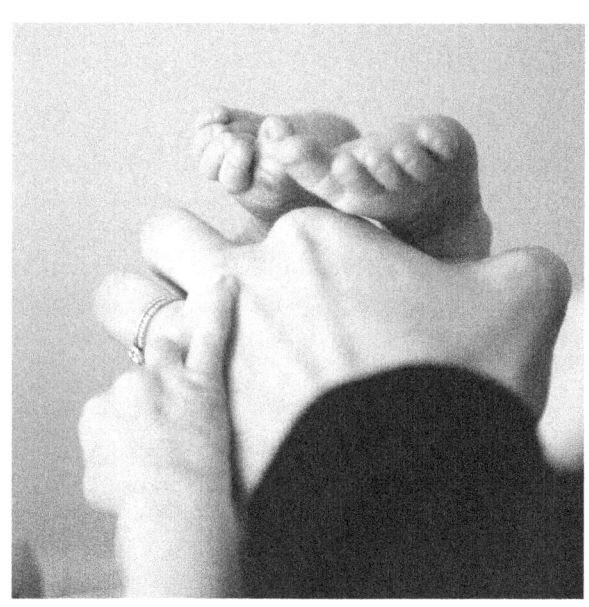

Paget

Paget disease of breast

Paget disease is uncommon, representing no more than 1 to 3 percent of new cases of female breast cancer. It is extremely rare among men. Paget disease is marked by a scaly or ulcerated lesion that starts on the nipple and then spreads to the areola. On occasion, a bloody nipple discharge may be present. Some patients will have associated pain, burning sensation, or itchiness.

An underlying breast cancer is present in 85 to 88 percent of cases, with a palpable mass associated in about half of cases. For 20 percent of patients, a non-palpable mammogram abnormality is present, while up to 15 percent of cases will not be linked to a palpable mass, mammogram abnormality, or any disease in the underlying breast tissue.

Initial evaluation
Your health care provider should obtain a detailed history, documenting the length of time the lesions has been present, associated symptoms. There should be an examination of both breasts.

What else could it be? Possibilities include benign causes such as eczema, a skin reaction to something, or nipple adenoma. Other cancer possibilities may include skin cancer. Given this range of diagnoses, a short course of steroids applied to the nipple and surrounding skin may be tried. Unfortunately, we sometimes see temporary improvement of the nipple and skin changes with such treatment, even if Paget disease is present. In this context, any persistent nipple abnormality should lead to a biopsy (tissue sampling).

Biopsy and imaging
Nipple scraping can accurately diagnosis Paget disease, but a so-called punch biopsy is usually done. The pathologist checks for estrogen and progesterone receptors, but about half of Paget disease cases will not have expression of these hormone receptors.

You need mammograms of both breasts, and an ultrasound should be used to further evaluate and guide biopsies of any mammogram-defined concerning lesion. Breast MRI may be added.

There are two theories to explain Paget disease of nipple:

- Epidermotropic theory (most accepted): Here, the Paget cell arises from an underlying breast cancer, with cells migrating through the ductal system into the nipple outer layer (epidermis).
- Transformation theory: The outer layer of cells of the nipple transform into malignant Paget cells; the Paget disease of nipple is independent of any underlying breast ductal cancer.

Management: Is there an underlying cancer?

The limited available evidence suggests that a central lumpectomy or complete resection of the nipple-areolar complex followed by whole breast radiation therapy is a reasonable approach for women with no palpable mass or mammogram abnormality. The surgical margins and cosmetic outcome should both be acceptable. A simple mastectomy is an alternative.

But what if you have Paget disease an there is an underlying cancer in the breast, too? Many patients will require a mastectomy, but if breast-conserving surgery of the nipple-areolar complex and the underlying cancer can be achieved with acceptable margins and cosmetic outcome, breast conserving surgery followed by whole breast radiation therapy may be offered. Those with cancer in several areas of the underlying breast (multicentri disease) or diffuse calcifications should have a mastectomy.

Axillary nodes

Those with pure ductal carcinoma *in situ* (DCIS or intraducatal carcinoma) do not need an evaluation of the nodes, although if you have a mastectomy, a limited (sentinel) sampling is routinely done. On the other hand anyone with invasive disease is generally recommended to have removal of a limited number of axillary nodes, irrespective of the surgery type. I think it is reasonable to do a sentinel node on anyone with Paget disease, in the chance that we find an unexpected invasive breast cancer during evaluation of the tissue after it is removed, although there is no consensus about this.

Systemic therapy is administered according to the cancer stage of the cancer. Women with Paget's disease treated with breast conservation (and radiation therapy) and without an associated cancer, or those with associated estrogen receptor-positive DCIS should consider endocrine therapy such as tamoxifen. Those with an associated invasive cancer should receive systemic therapy (some may need chemotherapy, for example) based on their risk of distant spread.

Young

Most breast cancers are found in women who are 50 years old or older, but breast cancer also affects younger women. **About 11% of all new cases of breast cancer in the United States are found among women younger than 45 years of age.** While breast cancer diagnosis and treatment are difficult for women of any age, young survivors may find it particularly overwhelming.

Get informed

Breast cancer in young women is —

- More likely to be hereditary than breast cancer in older women.
- More likely to be found at a later stage, and is often more aggressive and difficult to treat.
- Often coupled with unique issues, including concerns about body image, fertility, finances, and feelings of isolation.
- All women are at risk for getting breast cancer, but some things can raise a woman's risk for getting breast cancer before age 45.

If you are under the age of 45, you may have a higher risk for breast cancer if—

- You have close relatives who were diagnosed with breast cancer before the age of 45 or ovarian cancer at any age, especially if more than one relative was diagnosed or if a male relative had breast cancer.
- You have changes in certain breast cancer genes (BRCA1 and BRCA2), or have close relatives with these changes, but have not been tested yourself.
- You have Ashkenazi Jewish heritage.
- You received radiation therapy to the breast or chest during childhood or early adulthood.
- You have had breast cancer or certain other breast health problems, such as lobular carcinoma in situ (LCIS), ductal carcinoma in situ (DCIS), atypical ductal hyperplasia, or atypical lobular hyperplasia. You have been told that you have dense breasts on a mammogram.
- Do any of these characteristics describe you? If so, talk to your doctor about your family history and other risk factors you might have.

National Comprehensive Cancer Network, 2019 guidance

- **Inform:** All premenopausal patients should be informed about the potential impact of chemotherapy on fertility and asked about their desire for potential future pregnancies. Those who may desire future pregnancies should be referred to fertility specialists before chemotherapy and/or endocrine therapy to discuss the options based on patient specifics, disease stage, and biology (which determine the urgency and type and sequence of treatment).

- Although lack of menstrual periods frequently occurs during or after chemotherapy, it appears that the majority of women younger than 35 years resume menses within 2 years of finishing adjuvant chemotherapy.

- **Menses and fertility are not necessarily linked.** Absence of regular menses, particularly if the patient is taking tamoxifen, does not necessarily imply lack of fertility. Conversely, the presence of menses does not guarantee fertility. There are limited data regarding continued fertility after chemotherapy.

- **Patients should not become pregnant during treatment** with radiation therapy, or endocrine therapy.

- **Hormone-based birth control is discouraged** regardless of the hormone receptor status of the patient's cancer, although data is limited.

- **Alternative methods of birth control** include intrauterine devices (IUDs), barrier methods, or, for patients with no intent of future pregnancies, tubal ligation or vasectomy for the partner.

- **Breast feeding** following breast-conserving cancer treatment is not contraindicated. However, the quantity and quality of breast milk produced by the breast conserved may not be sufficient or may be lacking some of the nutrients needed. Breast feeding during active treatment with chemotherapy and endocrine therapy is not recommended.

Conception

For women with a history of breast cancer, a subsequent **pregnancy does not appear to compromise survival.** A 2012 study presented at the European Breast Cancer Conference suggests that pregnancy after breast cancer is safe, regardless of the estrogen receptor status. In addition, an analysis of a collection of 14 studies found that, compared with women who did not become pregnant, those sho became pregnant had a 40 percnt reduction in the risk of death. This advantage is probably the product of the "healthy mother effect": Only healthy survivors were able to conceive and carry a pregnancy.

For those who have received trastazumab (Herceptin), effective contraception should be used for at least seven months after stopping the drug before attempting pregnancy. The drug has been associated with fetal complications and even death.

Younger women may have chemotherapy-related infertility. Still others cannot try to conceive, as they are on endocrine therapy (for example, tamoxifen). We do not yet know the implications of interrupting endocrine therapy while attempting to conceive, but may get answers from the ongoing POSITIVE trial, a research study examining the feasibility of stopping endocrine therapy to have a child.

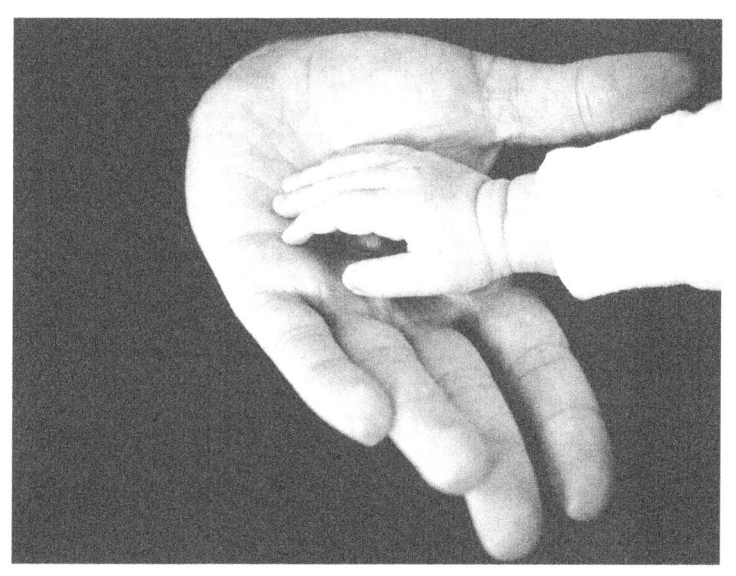

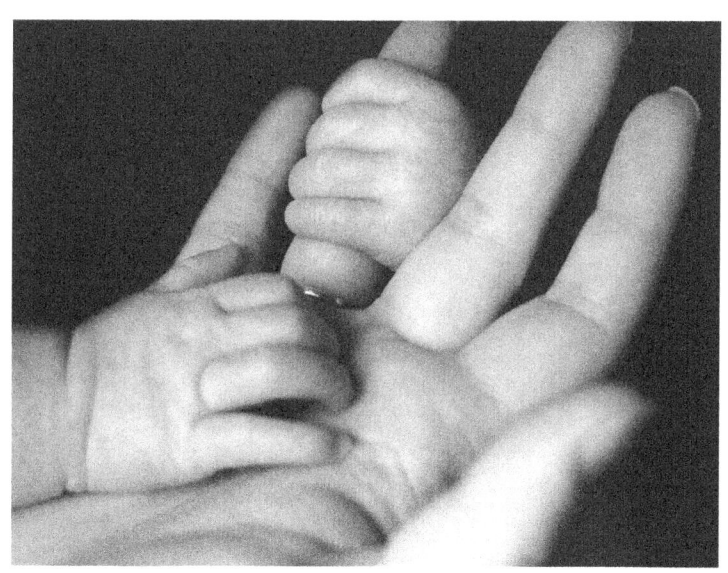

AFTER
Survivorship

Survivorship

DCIS

The National Comprehensive Cancer Network (NCCN), guidelines (version 1.2019) **ductal carcinoma *in situ* (DCIS)** call for:

• Consideration of endocrine therapy for 5 years for: 1) those treated with lumpectomy and radiation therapy (here, we have high-level evidence in support), especially for those with estrogen receptor positive DCIS. The benefits of endocrine therapy for ER negative DCIS is uncertain. Those who have lumpectomy alone (without radiation therapy) should also consider endocrine therapy.

• History and physical exam every 6 to 12 months for 5 years, then annually.

• Mammograms every 12 months (with the first one 6 to 12 months after breast-conserving therapy).

• For women on tamoxifen, annual gynecologic assessment (if uterus present)

• For women on an aromatase inhibitor, there should be monitoring of bone health with a bone mineral density (DEXA) test at baseline, and then periodically.

I would add the following:

• Encouragement of adherence to endocrine therapy (such as tamoxifen, or arotase inhibitor pills).

• Breast magnetic resonance imaging is not routinely recommended for breast cancer survivors. Still, breast MRI may be of value for patients suspected of having a breast cancer recurrence, or when the mammogram is inconclusive.

• Reconstructed breasts

For those who have had a breast removal or mastectomy, surveillance is primarily via physical examination.

Lifestyle

My patients frequently ask what they can do to optimize their prognosis from breast cancer. Lifestyle modification can be an effective and empowering way for not only help with physical and psychological well-being, but may improve your disease free- and overall survival opportunities.

Soy: Okay to eat

I am unaware of evidence to suggest that dietary soy (which contains phytoestrogens) affects breast cancer recurrence rates.

Alcohol: Increases risk

We do not have many studies linking alcohol consumption and with of recurremce. Still, the largest study showed that those who drank the equivalent of at least 3 to 4 standard drinks (more than 6 grams) of alcohol per week had significantly a 1.35-fold higher risk of recurrence and and 1.5-fold increase in breast cancer death, compared to those who consumed less tha 0.5 grams daily. The risk among overweight and postmenopausal women appeared highest, in this Life After Cancer Epidemiology (LACE) study.

Complementary

A comprehensive overview of this topic is beyond the scope of this book. The Society for Integrative Oncology (SIO) produced an evidence-based guideline on integrative therapies for the mangement of symptoms such as anxiety and stress, mood disorders, fatigue, chemotherapy-induced nausea and vomiting, lymphedema, chemotherapy-induced neuropathy, pain, and sleep disturbance.

The American Society of Clinical Oncology (ASCO) expert panel endorsed the guideline. Key recommendations include: Music therapy, meditation, stress management and yoga for anxiety and stress reduction. Meditation, relaxation, yoga, massage, and music therapy are recommended for depression/mood disorders. Meditation and yoga are recommended to improve quality of life. Acupressure and acupuncture are recommended for reducing chemotehrapy-induced nausea and vomiting. No strong evidence supports the use of ingested dietary supplements to manage breast cancer treatment-related side effects.

Physical activity, body weight, and diet

Observational studies show an association between survival and physical activity, with most of the data involveing patients with breast, colon, or prostate cancer.

Physical activity: Drops death rates

A meta-analysis of 16 prospective observational trials showed a near halving (48 percent reduction) in overall mortality and a 28 percent drop in breast cancer mortality in the most versus least active breast cancer survivors. Breast cancer survivors who increased their activity after diagnosis (relative to pre-diagnosis levels) dropped their mortality by more than a third (39 percent relative risk reduction).

Exercise can also help improve aerobic fitness, quality of life, strength, anxiety and depression, fatigue, body image, and body size and composition. It is not clear what the best exercise type is, but many of my patients aim for moderate activity such as a brisk walk for 30 minutes, five days per week.

Weight loss

Two large trials have looked at the benefits of weight loss among women with breast cancer. The Lifestyle Intervention Study for Adjuvant Treatment of Early Breast Cancer (LISA) randomly assigned 338 post-menopausal women with hormone receptor-positive breast cancer to a two-year telephone-based weight loss intervention or to usual care. The telephone group lost 5.4 percent weight by one year, and 3.7 percent at two years. The control group lost less (0.7 and 0.4 percent, respectively). In addition, those in the intervention group signifacntly improved their physical functioning. The Exercise and Nutrition to Enhance Recovery and Good Health for You (ENERGY) trial confirmed these results. We look forward to determining whether such weight loss improves breast cancer outcomes, as there are a number of trials looking at that.

Hot flashes

We generally avoid estrogen and progesterone for thise with a history of breast cancer. Some patients with severe symptoms may benefit from non-hormonal drugs suh as gabapentin in the evening or so-called serotonin reuptake inhibitors (SSRIs)/serotonin norepinephrine reuptake inhibitors (SNRIs). Some have concerns about interactions with tamoxifen, however. In this context, many avoid paroxetine or fluoxetine, but may use other drugs such as citalopram or venlafaxine.

Acupuncture has shown promising results in some clinical trials, with one study showing it works better than the drug gabapentin. A Wake Forest Baptist Medical Center (USA) study found that acupuncture reduced hot flashes and night sweats by over a third, with this benefit lasting for at least six months.

Depression and libido

Depression is a common result of breast cancer management, and can in turn affect sexuality. If you are depressed, please let your care team know. Many patients turn to therapists or group support. Antidepressant medications are sometimes offered, but this needs to be done in consultaton with your medical oncologist; some medicines may affect drugs such as tamoxifen. For example, paroxetin (Paxil), buprorion (Wellbutrin), Prozac, duloxetine (Cymbalta) and Zoloft may challenge your body's ability to convert tamoxifen into its active form, potentially reducing the full benefits of tamoxifen.

If loss of libido is an issue for you, you may be a candidate for testosterone (the primary hormone in men). However, if your testosterone levels are within normal limits, more testosterone will not likely provide a benefit to you. Finally, treatment-induced nausa can understandably take away your interest in sex.

Vaginal dryness

Menopause, whether natural or treatment-caused, may result in thinning and shortening of your vaginal walls. There can be associated dryness, or lack of lubrication which can lead to pain associated with sex. Some find relief with topical lidocaine. The American Society of Clinical Oncology recommends the use of non-hormonal treatments, including water- or silicone based lubricants of moisturizers as first line treatment for vaginal dryness and pain associated with sex. Vaginal moisturers include products containing gelatins, gums, polycarbophil, or hyaluronic acid.

Lymphedema (arm swelling)

Lymphedema (edema) is defined as the collection of protein-rich fluid in the spaces within a tissue, due disruption of the flow of lymph fluid. Lymphedema is an overflow problem: The lymph load exceeds the transport capacity of the lymphatic system. Unfortunately, this swelling (for example of the arm) can be associated with surgery or radiation therapy. It can manifesst as slowly progressive swelling of the arm, and can also include the breast or upper chest wall.

In a systematic review of 72 studies, the overall incidence of arm edema among survivors of breast cancer was 17 percent. Risk factors for breast cancer-associated lymphedema (arm swelling) include the following:

> **Axillary node dissecton**
> The surgical removal of nodes is the primary cause of breast and arm swelling, with the incidence increasing with the number of axillary

nodes removed or disrupted. The risk is around 20 percent for those who have an axillary node dissection (removal of several nodes from a grographic zone), compared to 5.6 percent for thos having a senting node biopsy.

Other

Excessive body weight (body mass index) can increase edema risk, as can infections after surgery, blood or fluid collections after surgery, and possibly medications such as chemotherapy. Weight gain can put you at additional risk, as it may impair lymphatic function.

The breast cancer management type may affect the timing of the development of lymphedema. It appears that early-onset edema (less than one year after surgery) may be more associated with surgery, while late-onset lymphedema seems more associated with radiation therapy to regional lyph nodes (note: patients who get radiation therapy for DCIS have more limited targets).

Lymphedema risk reduction

Primary prevention

The judicious use of a sentinel node sampling) rather than a more thorough axillary node dissection) is a primary means of reducing risk, but is not needed for most patients with DCIS. Sophisticated radiotherapy techniques may lower risk, too, as may surgical techniques such as reverse mapping or lymphatic bypass.

Secondary prevention

Here, the goal is to control arm swelling. We often monitor arm circumference. I ask patients to maintain excellent skin and nail care, as infection can lead to skin inflammation (cellulitis). A good skin mositurizer may help, as can protection of your hands with gloves when you are participating in activities that may lead to skin injury. If you have any signs of infection, report them.

Summary

DCIS

- **Excellent outcomes**

The 20-year disease-specific survival odds are 97%.

- **Improving outcomes**

The medical management of ductal carcinoma *in situ* in the USA keeps improving. The 5-year recurrence rate dropped from 13.6% to 6.6% when comparing lumpectomy-based results in the 1978 to 1998 period with 1999 to 2010).

- **Local therapy**

Surgery goes first (lumpectomy versus mastectomy). Then strong consideration should be given to radiation therapy for those who had had a breast-conserving surgery (no radiation therapy is an alternative approach). Those who have a mastectomy may consider breast reconstruction. Reconstruction can be immediate or delayed.

- **Systemic therapy**

Risk reduction therapy (such as tamoxifen (or an aromatase inhibitor for postmenopausal women) should be considered for patients managed with lumpectomy. The benefit for estrogen receptor-negative (ER-) DCIS remains uncertain. There should also be counseling regarding risk reduction strategies for the opposite breast.

- **Clear margins are important**

The local recurrence rate (even with radiation therapy) is as high as 20% if the margins are involved.

- **Gene testing**

Those at high-risk for hereditary breast cancer should have genetic counseling and consideration of genetic testing.

www.newcancerinfo.com

Final thoughts

by Michael Hunter MD

Thank you for allowing me to enter your life with this book. I hope that it has been valuable to you. Herein, I have tried to be clear in presenting information critical to you:

As we close, I ask that you too pursue, wherever possible, management strategies that are evidence-based. In this way, you optimize the chances of having the best care, while reducing your chances of potential harm. Now that we have addressed treatment, what can you do that may reduce your chances for a return (or progression) of the cancer?

- Have a balanced diet
- Optimize of your body:mass index
- Be prudent with alcohol consumption
- Try to be compliant with endocrine therapy, if you are on it.
- Avoid tobacco
- Get some physical activity

I wish you all the best, and feel privileged to communicate with you through this book. You may also find me at www.newcancerinfo.com. **Thank you!**

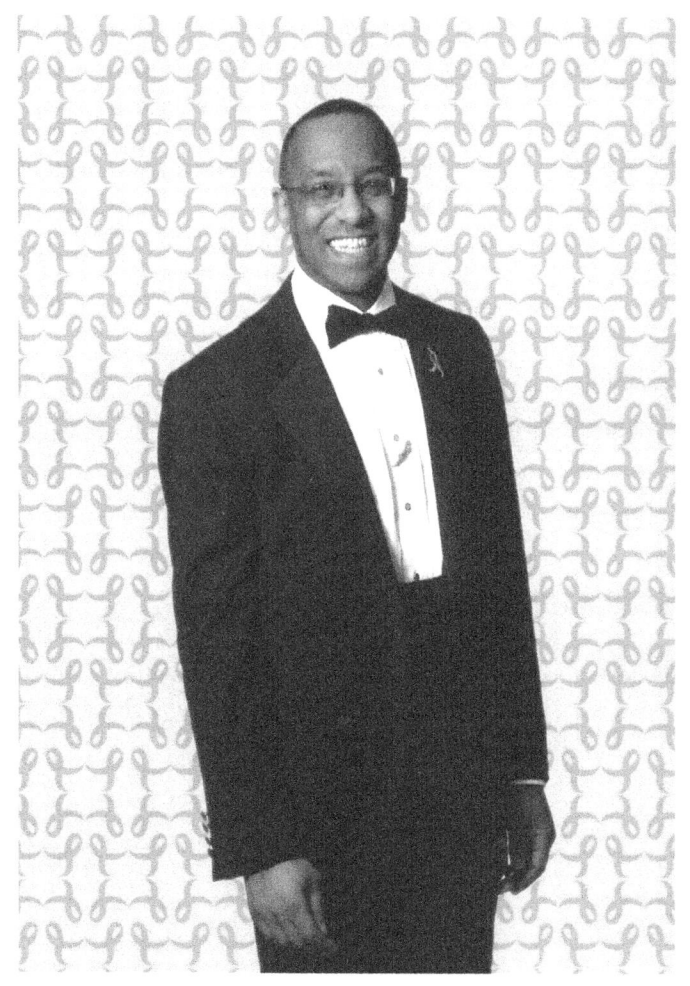

Thank you!

EDITING		Maya Hunter
IMAGES	p. 107	"Atypical ductal hyperplasia." Wikipedia. Wikipedia.org. n.p., en.wikipedia.org/wiki/Atypical_ductal_hyperplasia. Accessed 2 April 2019.
	p. 111	"Fibroadenoma." Wikipedia.org. n.p., en.wikipedia.org/wiki/Fibroadenoma. Accessed 2 April 2019.
		"Radial scar of breast - low mag.jpg." Wikimedia Commons, the free media repository. 20 Feb 2017, 17:38 UTC. Accessed 3 Apr 2019, commons.wikimedia.org/w/index.php?title=File:Radial_scar_of_breast_-_low_mag.jpg&oldid=234515060>.
	p. 113	"Phyllodes tumor." Wikipedia. Wikipedia.org. n.p., https://en.wikipedia.org/wiki/Phyllodes_tumor. Accessed 2 April 2019.
	p. 115	"Fat necrosis." Wikipedia. Widipedia.org. n.p., en.wikipedia.org/wiki/Fat_necrosis. Accessed 2 April 2019.
	p. 117	"Pseudoangiomatous stromal hyperplasia, abbreviated PASH. commons.wikimedia.org/w/index.php?search=Stromal+hyperplasia&title=Special%3ASearch&go=Go&ns0=1&ns6=1&ns12=1&ns14=1&ns100=1&ns106=1#/media/File:Pseudoangiomatous_stromal_hyperplasia_-a-_low_mag.jpg. Wikimedia. Wikimedia.org. Accessed 3 April 2019.
	p. 91; 193	Illustrations by Sarah Mahoney Voccola.
	p. 119	"Paget's disease of the breast." Wikipedia. Wikipedia.org. n.p., en.wikipedia.org/wiki/Paget%27s_disease_of_the_breast. Accessed 3 April 2019.
	p. 121	"Paget disease of the nipple." Wikimedia. commons.wikimedia.org/w/index.php?curid=9766336. Accessed 3 April 2019.

NOTES

1 basics

1. http://www.cancer.org/acs/groups/content/@editorial/documents/document/acspc-044552.pdf
2. http://globocan.iarc.fr/Pages/fact_sheets_cancer.aspx, 2014.
3. Stanford, J., Herrinton, L., Schwartz, S., & Weiss, N. (1995). Breast cancer incidence in Asian migrants to the United States and their descendants. Epidemiology, 6, 181–183.
4. Hemminki, K., & Li, X. (2002). Cancer risks in second-generation immigrants to Sweden. Int J Cancer, 99, 229–237.
5. Beiki, O., Hall, P., Ekbom, A., & Moradi, T. (2012). Breast cancer incidence and case fatality among 4.7 million women in relation to social and ethnic background: a population-based cohort study. Breast Cancer Res, 14(1), R5.
6. https://www.cancer.org/research/cancer-facts-statistics/breast-cancer-facts-figures.html

Age
7. American Cancer Society, Inc., Surveillance Research, 2017
8. http://www.targetedonc.com/news/expert-examines-impact-of-age-on-prognosis-molecular-subtype-in-breast-cancer

Race
9. CA: A Cancer Journal for Clinicians. doi: 10.3322/caac.21320. Online at cacancerjournal.com.
10. Keenan T, Moy B, Mroz EA, et al. Comparison of the Genomic Landscape Between Primary Breast Cancer in African American Versus White Women and the Association of Racial Differences With Tumor Recurrence. Presented at the 37th Annual San Antonio Breast Cancer Symposium, San Antonio, TX, December 9-13, 2014, and the 51st Annual Meeting of the American Society of Clinical Oncology, Chicago, IL, May 29-June 2, 2015.
11. American Cancer Society. Cancer Prevention & Early Detection Facts & Figures, 2015-2016.

Genes
12. http://www.cancer.gov/cancertopics/pdq/genetics/breast-and-ovarian/HealthProfessional#sthash.f98eeZ90.dpuf
13. Cancer (2015; doi: 10.1002/cncr.29645)
14. CA Cancer J Clin 2015
15. Walsh T, King MC. Ten genes for inherited breast cancer. Cancer Cell 2007; 11:103-5.
16. Hwang SJ, Lozano G, Amos CI et al. Germline p53 mutations ina cohort with chilhood sarcoma: sex differences in cancer risk. Am J Hum Genet 2003; 72(4):975-83.
17. Mouchawar J, Korch C, Byers T et al. Population-based estimate of the contribution of TP53 mutations to subgroups of early-onset breast cancer: Australian Breast Cancer Family Study. Cancer Res 2010; 70(12): 4705-800.
18. Melhem-Bertrandt A, Bojadzieva J, Ready KJ, et al. Early onset HER2-positive breast cancer is associated with germline TP53 mutations. Cancer 2012; 118(4): 908-13.
19. Min-Han T, Mester JL, Ngeow J, et al. Lifetime cancer risks in individuals with germline PTEN mutations. Clin Cancer Res 2012; 18(2): 400-7.
20. Walsh T, King MC. Ten genes for inherited breast cancer. Cancer Cell 2007; 11:103-5.

Radiation exposure
21. Land CE, Tokunaga M, Koyama K et al. Incidence of female breast cancer among atomic bomb survivors. Hiroshima and Nagasaki, 1950-1990. Radiat Res 2003;160: 707-717.
22. Preston DL, Mattsson A, Holmberg E et al. Radiation effects on breast cancer risk for young women treated for Hodgkin lymphoma. J Natl Cancer Inst 2005; 97:1428-37.

Family
23. Collaborative Group on Hormonal Factors in Breast Cancer: Familial breast cancer collaborative reanalysis of individual data from 52 epidemiological studies including 58,209 women with breast cancer and 101,986 women without the disease. Lancet 358: 1389-99, 2001.

Breast density
24. McCormack VA, dos Santos Silva I. Breast density and parenchymal patterns as markers of breast cancer risk: a meta-analysis. Cancer Epidemiol Biomarkers Prev. 2006;15:1159-1569
25. Katavic N, et al "Association of breast density with breast cancer risk in screening mammography" RSNA Meeting 2015; Abstract BR-5A-01.

Menarche, menopause, height, and obesity
26. Ritte R, et al. Height, age at menarche and risk of hormone receptor-positive and =negative breast cancer as a cohort study. Int J Cancer 2013; 132:2619.
27. Hsieh CC, et al. Age at menarche, age at menopause, height and obesity as risk factors for breast cancer: associations and interactions in an international case-control study. Int J Cancer 1990; 46:796.
28. Collaborative Group on Hormonal Factors in Breast Cancer. Menarche, menopause, and breast cancer risk: individual participant meta-analysis, including 118 964 women with breast cancer from 117 epidemiological studies. Lancet Oncol. 13(11):1141-51, 2012.
29. Colditz GA, et al. Cumulative risk of breast cancer to age 70 years according to risk factor status: data from the Nurses' Health Study. Am J Epidemiol 200; 152:950.

Childbearing; breast-feeding
30. Kelsey JL, et al. Reproductive factors and breast cancer. Epidemiol Rev 1993; 15:36.
31. Rosner B, et al. Reproductive risk factors in a prospective study of breast cancer: the Nurses' Health Study. Am J Epidemiol 1994; 139:814.
32. Annals of Oncology 00: 1–10, 2015 doi:10.1093/annonc/mdv379

Immigrants
33. John EM, Phipps AI, Davis A, Koo J. Migration history, acculturation, and breast cancer risk in Hispanic women. Cancer Epidemiol Biomarkers Prev 2005; 14:2905-13.

Alcohol
34. Alcohol drinking. IARC Working Ggroup, Lyon, 13-20 October 1987. IARC Mongr Eal Carcinog Risks Hum. 1988; 44:1-378.
35. Roswall N, Weiderpass E. Alcohol as a risk factor for cancer: existing evidence in a global perspective. J Prev Med Public Health. 2015; 48:1-9.

Weight gain
36. Newhouser ML et al. JAMA Oncol. 2015;doi:10.1001/jamaoncol.2015.1546.

Risk: Putting it all together (table)
37. Clemons M, et al. N Engl J Med 2001; 344: 276.

Diet
38. Estefania T, Salas-Salvado J, Donat-Vargas C, et al. Mediterranean diet and invasive breast cancer risk among women at high cardiovascular risk in the PREDIMED 10.1001.jamainternmed.2015.4838
39. Nutr Rev. 2014 Jan;72(1):1-17. doi: 10.1111/nure.12083. Epub 2013 Dec 13.
40. https://www.asco.org/about-asco/press-center/news-releases/balanced-low-fat-diet-reduces-risk-death-breast-cancer

Exposure to light (especially blue light)
41. http://www.health.harvard.edu/staying-healthy/blue-light-has-a-dark-side

Diabetes
42. A. S. Glicksman and R. W. Rawson, "Diabetes and altered carbohydrate metabolism in patients with cancer.," Cancer, vol. 9, no. 6, pp. 1127–34.
43. E. Giovannucci, D. M. Harlan, M. C. Archer, R. M. Bergenstal, S. M. Gapstur, L. a Habel, M. Pollak, J. G. Regensteiner, and D. Yee, "Diabetes and cancer: a consensus report.," Diabetes Care, vol. 33, no. 7, pp. 1674–85, Jul. 2010.
44. P. J. Hardefeldt, S. Edirimanne, and G. D. Eslick, "Diabetes increases the risk of breast cancer: a meta-analysis.," Endocr. Relat. Cancer, vol. 19, no. 6, pp. 793–803, Dec. 2012.
45. P. Boyle, M. Boniol, A. Koechlin, C. Robertson, F. Valentini, K. Coppens, L.-L. Fairley, T. Zheng, Y. Zhang, M. Pasterk, M. Smans, M. P. Curado, P. Mullie, S. Gandini, M. Bota, G. B. Bolli, J. Rosenstock, and P. Autier, "Diabetes and breast cancer risk: a meta-analysis.," Br. J. Cancer, vol. 107, no. 9, pp. 1608–17, Oct. 2012.
46. Centers for Disease Control and Prevention, "National diabetes fact sheet," 2011.

Thyroid cancer and breast cancer link
47. Hyun JA, Yul, H, Young AH, et al. A possible association between thyroid cancer and breast cancer. Thyroid. Dec 2015, 25(12):1330-1338.

Alcohol
48. Schütze M et al. Alcohol attributable burden of incidence of cancer in eight European countries based on results from prospective cohort study. BMJ. 2011 Apr 7;342:d1584.
49. https://www.pennmedicine.org/news/news-releases/2014/july/new-study-shows-drinking-alcoh

Triple negative breast cancer
50. Swain S. Triple-Negative Breast Cancer: Metastatic risk and role of platinum agents 2008 ASCO Clinical Science Symposium 2008. June 3, 2008.
51. Trivers KF, Lund MJ, Porter PL et al. The epidemiology of triple-negative breast cancer, including race. Cancer Causes Control 2009; 20: 1071.

Reproductive risk factors
52. Carey LA, Perou CM, Livasy CA, et al. Race, breast cancer subtypes, and survival in the Carolina Breast Cancer Study. JAMA 2006; 295:2492.
53. Phipps AI, Chlebowski RT, Prentice R, et al. Reproductive history and oral contraceptive use in relation to risk of triple-negative breast cancer. J Natl Cancer Inst 2011; 103: 470.
54. Phipps AI, Chlebowski RT, Prentice R, et al. Reproductive history and oral contraceptive use in relation to risk of triple-negative breast cancer. J Natl Cancer Inst 2011; 103: 470.
55. Anderson KN, Schwab RB, Martinez ME. Reproductive risk factors and breast cancer subtypes: a systmatic review of the literature. Breast Cancer Res Treat 2014; 144: 1.

56. Pierobon M, Frenkenfeld CL. Obseity as a risk factor for triple-negative breast caners: a systematic review and meta-analysis. Breast Cancer Res Treat 2013; 137: 307.
57. Palmer JR, Viscidi E, Troester MA, et al. Parity, lactation, andbreast cancer subtypes in African American women: results from the AMBER Consortium. J Natl Cancer Inst 2014; 106.

Breast cancer subtypes

58. Gonzalez-Angulo AM, Timms KM, et al. Incidence and outcome of BRCA mutations in unselected patients with triple receptor-negative breast cancer. Clin Cancer Res 2011; 17: 1082.
59. Millikan RC, Newman B, Tse CK, et al. Epidemioloy of basal-like breast cancer. Breast Cancer Res Treat 2008; 109:123.
60. Parise CA, Bauer KR, Brown MM, et al. Breast cancer subtypes as defined by the estrogen receptor (ER), progesterone receptor (PR), and the human epidermal growth factor receptor 2 (HER2) among women with invasive breast cancer in California, 1999-2004. Breast J 2009; 15: 593.

Male breast cancer

61. cancer.org/cancer/breastcancerinmen/detailedguide/breast-cancer-in-men-risk factors
62. cancer.org/cancer/breastcancerinmen/detailedguide/breast-cancer-in-men-risk-factors

Exposure to radiation

63. Land CE, Tokunaga M, Koyama K et al. Incidence of female breast cancer among atomic bomb survivors. Hiroshima and Nagasaki, 1950-1990. Radiat Res 2003;;160: 707-717.
64. Preston DL, Mattsson A, Holmberg E et al. Radiation effects on breast cancer risk for young women treated for Hodgkin lymphoma. J Natl Cancer Inst 2005; 97:1428-37.

Tobacco

65. Gaudet MM, Gapstur SM, Sun J, et al. Active smoking and breast cancer risk: original cohort data and meta-analysis. J Natl Cancer Inst. 105(8):515-25, 2013.
66. Dossus L, Boutron-Ruault MC, Kaaks R, et al. for the European Prospective Investigation into Cancer and Nutrition (EPIC) cohort. Active and passive cigarette smoking and breast cancer risk: results from the EPIC cohort. Int J Cancer. 134(8):1871-88, 2014.
67. Xue F, Willett WC, Rosner BA, Hankinson SE, Michels KB. Cigarette smoking and the incidence of breast cancer. Arch Intern Med. 171(2):125-133, 2011.
68. Hamajima N, Hirose K, Tajima K, et al. for the Collaborative Group on Hormonal Factors in Breast Cancer. Alcohol, tobacco and breast cancer--collaborative reanalysis of individual data from 53 epidemiological studies, including 58,515 women with breast cancer and 95,067 women without the disease. Br J Cancer. 87(11):1234-45, 2002.
69. Macacu A, Autier P, Boniol M, Boyle P. Active and passive smoking and risk of breast cancer: a meta-analysis. Breast Cancer Res Treat. 154(2):213-24, 2015.

"Preventative" Breast Removal

70. Newman LA ed. Surgical Oncology Clinics of North America, 2014; vol 23 (3).

DES

71. Howlader N, Noone AM,, Krapcho M, et al. (eds.) SEER Cancer Statistics Review, 1975-2009 (Vintage 2009 Populations), National Cancer Institute. Bethesda, MD, 2012. Retrieved April 25, 2017.

Risk calculators; risk reduction
72. http://ccge.medschl.cam.ac.uk/boadicea/ Centre for Cancer Genetic Epidemiology. BOADI-CEA. Accessed March 14, 2017.
73. http://www.ems-trials.org/riskevaluation/ Accessed March 14, 2017.
74. https://www.cancer.gov/bcrisktool/ Accessed March 14, 2017.
75. http://www.yourdiseaserisk.wustl.edu/ Siteman Cancer Center. Accessed March 14, 2017.
76. Goss PR, Ingle JN, Pritchard K, et al: Extending aromatase-inhibitor therapy to 10 years. N Engl J Med 375:209-219, 2016.
77. Chlebowski R. Improving Breast Cancer Risk Assessment Versus Implementing Breast Cancer Prevention. J Clin Oncol, 35(7), 2017: 702-704.
78. Newman L and Petrelli N, eds. Breast cancer. Surgical Oncology Clinics of North America 23 (3): 424-425, 2014.
79. DeCensi A, Puntoni M, Guerrieri-Gonzaga A et al. Randomized placebo controlled trial of low-dose tamoxifen to prevent local and contralateral recurrence in breast intraepithelial neoplasia. J Clin Oncol 37 (19):1629-1637. 2019.

Oral contraceptives
80. Collaborative Group on Hormonal Factors in Breast Cancer. Breast cancer and hormonal contraceptives: collaborative reanalysis of individual data on 53,297 women with breast cancer and 100,239 women without breast cancer from 54 epidemiological studies. Collaborative Group on Hormonal Factors in Breast Cancer. Lancet. 347:1713-27, 1996.
81. Gierisch JM, Coeytaux RR, Urrutia RP, et al. Oral contraceptive use and risk of breast, cervical, colorectal, and endometrial cancers: a systematic review. Cancer Epidemiol Biomarkers Prev. 22(11):1931-43, 2013.

Breast feeding
82. Collaborative Group on Hormonal Factors in Breast Cancer. Breast cancer and breast feeding: collaborative reanalysis of individual data from 47 epidemiological studies in 30 countries, including 50,302 women with breast cancer and 96,973 women without the disease. Lancet 20:187-95, 2002. - See more at: http://ww5.komen.org/BreastCancer/LowerYourRiskReferences.html#sthash.XMUSDrLo.dpuf

Hormone replacement therapy
83. Goss PE, Ingle JN, Alés-Martínez JE, et al. for the NCIC CTG MAP.3 Study Investigators. Exemestane for breast-cancer prevention in postmenopausal women. N Engl J Med. 364(25):2381-91, 2011.
84. U.S. Food and Drug Administration. Menopause and hormones: Common questions. http://www.fda.gov/ForConsumers/ByAudience/ForWomen/ucm118624.htm, 2014.
85. Holmberg L, Iverson OE, Rudenstam CM, et al., for the HABITS Study Group. Increased risk of recurrence after hormone replacement therapy in breast cancer survivors. J Natl Cancer Inst. 100(7):475-82, 2008.
86. Colditz GA, Hankinson SE, Hunter DJ, et al. The use of estrogens and progestins and the risk of breast cancer in postmenopausal women. N Engl J Med. 332: 1589-93, 1995.
87. Cancer Epidemiol Biomarkers Prev. 2005 Dec;14(12):2905-13.
Migration history, acculturation, and breast cancer risk in Hispanic women.
88. John EM, Phipps AI, Davis A, Koo J. Cancer Epidemiol Biomarkers Prev. 2005 Dec;14(12):2905-13. Migration history, acculturation, and breast cancer risk in Hispanic women.

Worldwide - Incidence
89. https://www.wcrf.org/dietandcancer/cancer-trends/breast-cancer-statistics

2 image

Mammograms
1. U.S. Preventive Services Task Force. Ann Intern Med. 151(10):716-726, 2009.
2. http://www.cancer.org/cancer/breastcancer/moreinformation/breastcancerearlydetection/breast-cancer-early-detection-acs-rec
3. http://www.nccn.org/professionals/physician_gls/pdf/breast-screening.pdf

Age
4. NCI-funded Breast Cancer Surveillance Consortium (HHSN261210000031C) http://breasscreening.cancer.gov/ (Accessed on November 09, 2015).
5. Fletcher SW, Elmore JG. Clinical practice. Mammographic screening for breast cancer. N Engl J Med. 2003;348:1672-1680.
6. Schonberg MA, McCarthy EP, Davis RB, et al. Breast cancer screening in women aged 80 and older: results from a national survey. J Am Geriatr Soc. 2004;52:1688-1695.
7. Schonberg MA, Ramanan RA, McCarthy EP, Marcantonio ER. Decision making and counseling around mammography screening for women aged 80 or older. J Gen Intern Med. 2006;21:979-985.
Breast Tumor Prognostic Characteristics and Biennial vs Annual Mammography, Age, and Menopausal Status
8. Miglioretti DL, Zhu W, Kerlikowske K. Breast tumor prognostic characteristics and biennial vs annual mammography, age, and menopausal status. JAMA Oncol. 2015;1(8):1069-1077.

Mammograms: Cons
9. U.S. Preventive Services Task Force. Screening for breast cancer: U.S. Preventive Services Task Force recommendation statement. Ann Intern Med. 151(10):716-726, 2009.
10. Ronckers CM, Erdmann CA, Land CE: Radiation and breast cancer: a review of current evidence. Breast Cancer Res 7 (1): 21-32, 2005.
11. Goss PE, Sierra S: Current perspectives on radiation-induced breast cancer. J Clin Oncol 16 (1): 338-47, 1998.
12. Radiology 241 (1): 55-66, 2006.
13. Bleyer A, Welch HG: N Engl J Med 367 (21): 1998-2005, 2012.
14. Jørgensen KJ, Gøtzsche PC: BMJ 339: b2587, 2009.
15. Kalager M, Zelen M, Langmark F, et al.: N Engl J Med 363 (13): 1203-10, 2010.

Breast MRI
16. American College of Radiology. ACR Practice Parameter for the Performance of Contrast-Enhanced Magnetic Resonance Imaging (MRI) of the Breast. http://www.acr.org/~/media/2a0eb28eb59041e2825179afb72ef624.pdf. Accessed June 15, 2015.
17. Dontchos BN, DeMartini WB, Rahbar H, Peacock S, Lehman CD. Influence of Menstrual Cycle Timing on Screening Breast MRI Performance in Pre-Menopausal Women. Presented at: Radiological Society of North America (RSNA) Annual Meeting; November 25-30, 2012; Chicago, IL.
18. Saslow D et al. CA Cancer J Clin 2007;57:75-89

Ultrasound
19. Berg WA, Zhang Z, Lehrer D, et al. for the ACRIN 6666 Investigators. Detection of breast cancer with addition of annual screening ultrasound or a single screening MRI to mammography in women with elevated breast cancer risk. JAMA. 307(13):1394-404, 2012.
20. Scheel JR, Lee JM, Sprague BL, Lee CI, Lehman CD. Screening ultrasound as an adjunct to mammography in women with mammographically dense breasts. Am J Obstet Gynecol. 212(1):9-17. 2015.

Tomosynthesis
21. Skaane P, Bandos AI, Gullien R, et al. Comparison of digital mammography alone and digital mammography plus tomosynthesis in a population-based screening program. Radiology. 267(1):47-56, 2013.
22. Ciatto S, Houssami N, Bernardi D, et al. Integration of 3D digital mammography with tomosynthesis for population breast-cancer screening (STORM): a prospective comparison study. Lancet Oncol. S1470-2045(13)70134-7, 2013.
23. Friedewald SM, Rafferty EA, Rose SL, et al. Breast cancer screening using tomosynthesis in combination with digital mammography. JAMA. 311(24):2499-2507, 2014.
24. http://www.cancer.org/cancer/news/news/breast-cancer-screening-with-3-d-technology-finds-more-cancers
25. http://www.massgeneral.org/imaging/services/3D_mammography_tomosynthesis.aspx
High-risk: Screening
26. American Cancer Society. Mammogram reports – BI-RADS.
27. U.S. Preventive Services Task Force. Screening for breast cancer: U.S. Preventive Services Task Force recommendation statement. Ann Intern Med. 151(10):716-726, 2009.
28. http://www.facingourrisk.org/understanding-brca-and-hboc/publications/documents/Surveillance%20Flyer%207.16.14.pdf

Molecular imaging
29. Hendrick RE. Radiation doses and cancer risks from breast imaging studies. Radiology. 257(1):246-53, 2010.

Clinical breast exam
30. Fenton JJ, Rolnick SJ, Harris EL, et al.: Specificity of clinical breast examination in community practice. J Gen Intern Med 22 (3): 332-7, 2007.

Thermography
31. Lee CI and Elmore JC. Chap 11. Breast Cancer Screening, in Harris JR, Lippman ME, Morrow M, Osborne CK. Diseases of the Breast, 5th edition. Lippincott Williams and Wilkins, 2014.
32. http://www.fda.gov/NewsEvents/Newsroom/PressAnnouncements/ucm257633.htm

MRI
33. Berg WA, Zhang Z, Lehrer D, et al. for the ACRIN 6666 Investigators. Detection of breast cancer with addition of annual screening ultrasound or a single screening MRI to mammography in women with elevated breast cancer risk. JAMA. 307(13):1394-404, 2012.
34. Pinsky RW, Helvie MA. Mammographic breast density: effect on imaging and breast cancer risk. J Natl Compr Canc Netw. 8(10):1157-64, 2010.
35. O'Flynn EA, Ledger AE, deSouza NM. Alternative screening for dense breasts: MRI. AJR Am J Roentgenol. 204(2):W141-9, 2015.
36. Tagliafico AS, et al. Adjuvant scrrening with tomosynthesis or ultrasound in women with mammography-neagative dense breasts: Interim report of a prospective comparative trial. J Clin Oncol 34: 1883-88 (16), 2016.

Self-exam
37. Thomas DB, Gao DL, Ray RM, et al.: Randomized trial of breast self-examination in Shanghai: final results. J Natl Cancer Inst 94 (19): 1445-57, 2002.
38. Semiglazov VF, Manikhas AG, Moiseenko VM, et al.: [Results of a prospective randomized investigation [Russia (St.Petersburg)/WHO] to evaluate the significance of self-examination for the early detection of breast cancer]. Vopr Onkol 49 (4): 434-41, 2003.

Breast density; high risk imaging
39. Gierach GL, Ichikawa L, Kerlikowske K, et al. Relationship between mammographic density and breast cancer death in the Breast Cancer Surveillance Consortiu. J Natl Cancer Inst 2012; 104(16):1218-27.
40. https://www.breastcancer.org/symptoms/testing/types/mri/screening

Fact box
41. Gøtzsche PC, Jørgensen KJ (2013). Cochrane Database of Systematic Reviews (6): CD001877.pub5.
42. https://www.harding-cancer.mpg.de/en/health-information/facts-boxes/mammography

Inflammatory breast cancer
43. http://www.cancer.net/cancer-types/breast-cancer-inflammatory/statistics
44. Chow CK. Imaging in inflammatory breast carcinoma. Breast Dis 2005-2006;22:45–54.
45. Tardivon AA, Viala J, Corvellec Rudelli A, Guinebretiere JM, Vanel D. Mammographic patterns of inflammatory breast carcinoma: a retrospective study of 92 cases. Eur J Radiol 1997;24(2):124–130.

DCIS:Imaging
46. http://www.medscape.com/viewarticle/810492
47. Pilewskie M, et al. Ann Surg Oncol. 2014 May; 21(5): 1552–1560.
48. Dershaw DD, Abramson A, Kinne DW. Ductal carcinoma in sity: mammographic findings and clinical implications. Radiology 1989;170(2):411.

3 biopsy

DCIS
1. Bestill WL Jr., Rosen PP, Lieberman PH, Robbins GF. Intraductal carcinoma: long-term follow-up after treatment by biopsy alone. JAMA 1978;239(18):1863-1867. CrossRefMedlineWeb of ScienceGoogle Scholar
2. Eusebi V, Feudale E, Foschini MP, et al. Long-term follow-up of in situ carcinoma of the breast. Sem Diag Pathol 1994;11:223-235.
3. Page DL, Dupont WD, Rogers LW, Landenberger M. Intraductal carcinoma of the breast: follow-up after biopsy only. Cancer 1982;49(4):751-758.
4. Rosen PP, Braun DW Jr., Kinne DE. The clinical significance of preinvasive breast carcinomas. Cancer 1980;46:919-925.
5. Semin Diagn Pathol 1994;11:208–14.
6. http://www.breastcancer.org/symptoms/testing/types/biopsy
7. Wellings RR, Jensen HM. On the origin and progression of ductal carcinoma in the human breast. J Natl Cancer Inst 1973;50(5):1111-1118.

8. Cheatle GL, Cutler M. Malignant epithelial neoplasia. Carcinoma. The precancerous or potentially carcinomatous state. In: Cheatle GL, Cutler M, editors. Tumours of the Breast. 1st ed. Philadelphia, PA: Lippincott; 1926. p. 161-332.
9. Foote FW, Stewart FW. Comparative studies of cancerous versus noncancerous breasts. Ann Surg 1945;121(1):6-53. 197–222.
10. Page DL, Rogers LW. Carcinoma in situ (CIS). In: Page DL, Anderson TJ, editors. Diagnostic Histopathology of the Breast. 1st ed. New York, NY: Churchill Livingston; 1987. p. 157-174.
11. Wellings SR, Jensen HM, Marcum RG. An atlas of subgross pathology of the human breast with special reference to possible precancerous lesions. J Natl Cancer Inst 1975;55(2):231-273.
12. Muir R. The evolution of carcinoma of the mamma. J Pathol Bacteriol 1941;LII(2):155-172.
13. Fechner RE. History of ductal carcinoma in situ. In: Silverstein ML, editor. Ductal Carcinoma In Situ of the Breast. 2nd ed. Philadelphia, PA: Lippincott Williams and Wilkins; 2002. p. 3-16.
14. Rose RE, Paulson EC, Sharma A, et al. HER-2/neu overexpression as a predictor for the transition from in situ to invasive breast cancer. Cancer Epidemiol Biomarkers Prev 2009;18:1386-1389.

Benign breast disases
15. Hartmann LC, Degnim AC, Santen RJ, et al. N Engl J Med. 2015;372:78-89.
16. Hartmann LC, Radisky DC, Frost MH, et al. Cancer Prev Res (Phila). 2014;7:211-217.
17. Page DL, Schuyler PA, Dupont WD, et al. Lancet. 2003;361:125-129
18. Sabel MS. Overview of benign breast disease. In: Chagpar AB, ed. UpToDate. Waltham, MA, UpToDate, 2015.
19. https://en.wikipedia.org/wiki/Atypical_ductal_hyperplasia#/media/File:Atypical_ductal_hyperplasia_-_high_mag.jpg

DCIS versus LCIS
20. Mommers ER, et al. J Pathol 194:327-333.
21. Warnberg et al. Br J Cancer 85:869-874.
22. JAMA. 2015;313(11):1122-1132.

DCIS and HER2
23. Latta EK, Tain S, Parkes RK, O'Malley FP. The role of HER2/neu overexpression in the progression of ductal carcinoma in situ to invasive carcinoma of the breast. Mod Pathol 2002 Dec; 15(12):1318-25.

Microinvasion
24. Sue GR, Lannin DR. Killelea B, Chagpar AB. Predictors of microinvasion and its prognostic role in ductal carcinoma *in situ*. Am J Surg 2013; 206(4):478.
25. Vieirra CC, Mercado CL, Cangiarella JF, et al. Microinvasive ductal carcinoma in situ: clinical presentation, imaging features, pathologic findings, and outcome. Eur J Radiol. 2010 Jan;73(1):102-7.

26. Chen CY, Sun LM, Anderson BO. Paget disease of the breast: changing patterns of incidence, clinical presentation, and treatment in the U.S. Cancer 2006; 107(7):1448.
27. Ashikari R, Park K, Huvos AG, et al. Paget's disease of the breast. Cancer. 1970; 26(3):680.
28. Nance FC, DeLoach DH, Welsh RA, et al. Paget's disease of the breast. Ann Surg 1970; 171(6):864.
29. https://en.wikipedia.org/wiki/Paget%27s_disease_of_the_breast#/media/File:Extramammary_Paget_disease_-_high_mag.jpg

Fat necrosis
30. https://en.wikipedia.org/wiki/Fat_necrosis#/media/File:Breast_tissue_showing_fat_necrosis_4X.jpg

Margins
32. Moran MS, Stuart Schnitt J, Giuliano AE, et al. Society of Surgical Oncology–American Society for Radiation Oncology Consensus Guideline on Margins for Breast-Conserving Surgery With Whole-Breast Irradiation in Stages I and II Invasive Breast Cancer. Annals of Surgical Oncology; March 2014, Volume 21, Issue 3, pp 704-716.

Invasive ductal cancer
33. Li CI, Uribe DJ, Daling JR. Clinical characteristics of different histologic types of breast cancer. Br J Cancer 2005; 93: 1046.

HER2
34. Slamon DJ, Godolphin W, Jones LA, et al. Science. 1989;244:707-712.
35. Sliwkowski MX. In: Harris JR, Lippman ME, Morrow M, Osborne CK, eds. Diseases of the Breast. 3rd ed. Philadelphia, PA: Lippincott Williams & Wilkins; 2004:415-426.
36. Ménard S, Tagliabue E, Campiglio M, Pupa SM. J Cell Physiol. 2000;182:150-162.
37. Sergina NV, Rausch M, Wang D, et al. Nature. 2007;445:437-441.

Paget's disease of the nipple
38. Photomicrograph: https://en.wikipedia.org/wiki/Paget%27s_disease_of_the_breast
39. Thin G. On the connection between disease of the nipple and areola and tumors of the breast. Trans Pathol Soc Lond 1881; 32:218.
40. Morrow M, Harris JR. Ductal carcinoma in situ and microinvasive carcinoma. In: Harris JR, Lippman ME, Morrow M, Osborne CK, editors. Diseases of the Breast. 3rd ed. Philadelphia, PA: Lippincott Williams and Wilkins; 2004. p. 521-537.
41. http://jncimono.oxfordjournals.org/content/2010/41/134.long#ref-3
42. Semin Diagn Pathol 1994;11:208–14.
43. Lewis GD, Lofgren JA, McMurtrey AE, et al. Cancer Res. 1996;56:1457-1465.
44. http://www.gene.com/patients/disease-education/her2-disease-in-breast-cancer
45. http://ww5.komen.org/BreastCancer/SubtypesofBreastCancer.html#sthash.qOuPw8j5.dpuf
46. Moran MS, Stuart Schnitt J, Giuliano AE, et al. Society of Surgical Oncology–American Society for Radiation Oncology Consensus Guideline on Margins for Breast-Conserving Surgery With Whole-Breast Irradiation in Stages I and II Invasive Breast Cancer. Annals of Surgical Oncology 2014;21 (3): 704-716.

Phylloides
47. https://en.wikipedia.org/wiki/Phyllodes_tumor#/media/File:Phylloidestumor_der_Mamma_-_Mammographie.jpg

Intraductal papilloma; PASH
48. Sydnor MK et al. Underestimation of the presence of breast carcinoma in papillary lesions initially diagnosed at core-needle biopsy. Radiology 242 (1) 2007: 58-62.
https://en.wikipedia.org/wiki/Pseudoangiomatous_stromal_hyperplasia

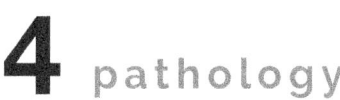

5 biopsy
6 chances: dcis
7-12 management

1. http://media.jamanetwork.com/news-item/study-examines-breast-cancer-mortality-after-ductal-carcinoma-in-situ-diagnosis/
2. National Comprehensive Cancer Network (NCCN). NCCN Clinical practice guidelines in oncology: Breast cancer v.3.2014, http://www.nccn.org/, 2014.
3. Wapnir IL, Dignam JJ, Fisher B, et al. Long-term outcomes of invasive ipsilateral breast tumor recurrences after lumpectomy in NSABP B-17 and B-24 randomized trials for DCIS. J Natl Cancer Inst 2011; 103:478.
4. Van Zee KJ, White J, Morrow M, Harris JR. Chapter 23: Ductal carcinoma in situ and microinvasive carcinoma. In Harris JR, Lippman ME, Morrow M, Osborne CK. Diseases of the Breast. 5th edition. Lippincott Williams and Wilkins, 2014.
5. Recht, A. Are the Randomized Trials of Radiation Therapy for Ductal Carcinoma in Situ Still Relevant? J Clin Oncol 32 (32), 2014.

Tamoxifen
6. Kane RL, Virnig BA, Shamliyan T, et al. The impact of surgery, radiation, and systemic treatment on outcomes in patients with ductal carcinoma in situ: a study based on NSABP protocol B-24. J Clin Oncol. 30(12):1268-73, 2012.
7. D. Craig Allred, Stewart J. Anderson, Soonmyung Paik, et al. Adjuvant tamoxifen reduces subsequent breast cancer in women with estrogen receptor-positive ductal carcinoma in situ: A study based on NSABP protocol B-24. J Clin Oncol. 2012 Apr 20; 30(12); 1268-73.
8. Wapnir IL, Dignam JJ, Fisher B, et al. Long-term outcomes of invasive ipsilateral breast tumor recurrences after lumpectomy in NSABP B-17 and B-24 randomized clinical trials for DCIS. J Natl Cancer Inst 2011;103:478-488.

Review of randomized trials
9. Goodwin A, Parker S, Ghersi D, Wilcken N. Post-operative radiotherapy for ductal carcinoma in situ of the breast - a systematic review of the randomised trials. Breast 2009; 18:143.

HER2 status
10. G. Curigliano, D. Disalvatore, A. Esposito et al. Risk of subseuqent in situ and invasive breast cancer in human epidermal growth factor receptor 2-positive ductal carcinoma in situ. Ann Oncol 2015;26(4):682-687.
11. Michael D Alvarado, Mitchell T Hayes, Rajni Sethi, Elissa Ozanne. NSABP B-43 is unlikely to produce a cost-effective treatment strategy for HER2+ DCIS [abstract]. In: Proceedings of the Thirty-Seventh Annual CTRC-AACR San Antonio Breast Cancer Symposium: 2014 Dec 9-13; San Antonio, TX. Philadelphia (PA): AACR; Cancer Res 2015;75(9 Suppl):Abstract nr P1-10-03.

Microinvasive carcinoma
12. Vieira CC, Mercado CL, Cangiarella JF et al. Microinvasive ductal carcinoma in sity: clinical presentation imaging features, pathologic findings, and outcome. Eur J Radiol 2010; 73(1): 102-107.
13. Padmore RF, Fowble B Hoffman J et al. Microinvasive breast carcinoma: clinicopathologic analysis of a single institution experience. Cancer 2000; 88(6): 1403-1409.
14. Adamovich TL, Simmons RM. Ductal carcinoma in situ with microinvasion. Am J Surg 2003; 186(2): 112-116.
15. Margalit DN, Sreedhara M, Chen YH, et al. Microinvasive breast cancer: ER, PR, and HER-2/neu status and clinical outcomes after breast-conserving therapy or mastectomy. Ann Surg Oncol 2013; 20(3):811-8.
16. Sue GR, Lannin DR, Killelea B, Chagpar AB. Predictors of microinvasion and its prognostic role in ductal carcinoma in situ. Am J Surg 2013; 206(4):478-88.
17. de Mascarel I, MacGrogan G, Mathoulin-Pelissier S, et al. Breast ductal carcinoma in situ with microinvasion: a definition supported by a long-term study of 1248 serially sectioned ductal carcinomas. Cancer 2002; 94(8):2134-2142.
18. Sue GR, Lannin DR, Killelea B, Chagpar AB. Predictors of microinvasion and its prognostic role in ductal carcinoma in situ. Am J Surg 2013; 206(4): 478.

Margins
19. Dunne C, Burke JP, Morrow M, Kell MR. Effect of margin status on local recurrence after breast conservation and radiation therapy for ductal carcinoma in situ. J Clin Oncol 2009; 27:1615-1620.
20. Groot G, Rees H, Pahwa P, et al. Predicting local recurrence following breast-consering therapy for early stage breast cancer: the significance of a narrow (</= 2mm) surgical resection margin. J Surg Oncol 2011; 103:212-216.
21. http://www.nccn.org
22. 2014 San Antonio Breast Cancer Symposium validated this gene test in a diverse population of women with DCIS (Abstract S5-04).
23. Moran MS, Stuart Schnitt J, Giuliano AE, et al. Society of Surgical Oncology–American Society for Radiation Oncology Consensus Guideline on Margins for Breast-Conserving Surgery With Whole-Breast Irradiation in Stages I and II Invasive Breast Cancer. Annals of Surgical Oncology; 2014, Volume 21, Issue 3, pp 704-716.

Molecular profiling
24. Hughes LL, Wang M, Page DL, et al. Local excision alone without irradiation for ductal carcinoma in situ of the breast: a trial of the Eastern Cooperative Oncology Group. J Clin Oncol 2009;27:5319-24.
25. JAMA Oncol. 2015 Oct;1(7):888-96. doi: 10.1001/jamaoncol.2015.2510. Breast Cancer Mortality After a Diagnosis of Ductal Carcinoma In Situ.

Locoregional recurrence
106. EBCTCG Lancet Oncol 378:1707-16, 2011

Mammograms
3. Gold RH, Bassett LW, Widoff BE. Highlights from the history of mammography. Radiographics 1990; 10(6):1111.
4. Muir BB, Kirkpatrick AE, Roberts MM et al. Oblique-view mammography: adequacy for screening. Work in progress. Radiology 1984;151(1);39.
5. Wald NJ, Murphy P, Major P et al. UKCCCR multicentre randomised controlled trial of one and two view mammography in breast cancer screening. BMJ 1995;311(7014):1189.

6. Ikeda DM, Andersson I. Radiology 1989;172(3):661.
7. Friedewald SM, Rafferty EA, Rose SL, et al. Breast cancer screening using tomosynthesis in combination with digital mammography. JAMA 2014;311(24):2499.

MRI
8. http://www.medscape.com/viewarticle/810492
9. Pilewskie M, Olcese C, BS,Eaton A et al. Perioperative Breast MRI Is Not Associated with Lower Locoregional Recurrence Rates in DCIS Patients Treated With or Without Radiation. Ann Surg Oncol. 2014 May; 21(5): 1552–1560.

Biopsy
10. Brennan ME, Turner RM, Clatto S et al. Ductal carcinoma in situ at core-needle biopsy: meta-analysis of underestimation and predictors of invasive breast cancer. Radiology 2011;260:119-128.
11. https://en.wikipedia.org/wiki/Paget%27s_disease_of_the_breast#/media/File:Extramammary_Paget_disease_-_high_mag.jpg

Management
12. Narod SA, Iqbal J, Giannakeas V, et al. Breast cancer mortality after a dignosis of ductal carcinoma in situ. JAMA Oncol 2015;1(7):888.
13. Rosner D, Bedwani RN, Vana J et al. Noninvasive breast carcinoma: results of a national survey by the American College of Surgeons. Ann Surg 1980;192(2):139.
14. Kinne DW, Petrek JA, Osborne MP et al. Breast carcinoma in situ. Arch Surg 1989;124(1):33.
15. Goodwin A, Parker S, Ghersi D, et al. Breast 2009;18(3):143.
16. Wapnir IL, Dignam JJ, Fisher B, et al: Long- term outcomes of invasive ipsilateral breast tumor recurrences after lumpectomy in NSABP B-17 and B-24 randomized clinical trials for DCIS. J Natl Cancer Inst 103:478-488, 2011
17. RT boost: JAMA Oncol. Published online March 30, 2017. doi:10.1001/jamaoncol.2016.6948

Mammograms
3. Gold RH, Bassett LW, Widoff BE. Highlights from the history of mammography. Radiographics 1990; 10(6):1111.
4. Muir BB, Kirkpatrick AE, Roberts MM et al. Oblique-view mammography: adequacy for screening. Work in progress. Radiology 1984;151(1);39.

13 special

Pregnancy-related breast cancer
1. Clark RM, Chua T: Breast cancer and pregnancy: the ultimate challenge. Clin Oncol (R Coll Radiol) 1 (1): 11-8, 1989.
2. Yang WT, Dryden MJ, Gwyn K, et al.: Imaging of breast cancer diagnosed and treated with chemotherapy during pregnancy. Radiology 239 (1): 52-60, 2006.
3. Middleton LP, Amin M, Gwyn K, et al.: Breast carcinoma in pregnant women: assessment of clinicopathologic and immunohistochemical features. Cancer 98 (5): 1055-60, 2003.
4. Middleton LP, Amin M, Gwyn K, et al.: Breast carcinoma in pregnant women: assessment of clinicopathologic and immunohistochemical features. Cancer 98 (5): 1055-60, 2003.
5. Elledge RM, Ciocca DR, Langone G, et al.: Estrogen receptor, progesterone receptor, and HER-2/neu protein in breast cancers from pregnant patients. Cancer 71 (8): 2499-506, 1993.

6. Petrek JA, Dukoff R, Rogatko A: Prognosis of pregnancy-associated breast cancer. Cancer 67 (4): 869-72, 1991.
7. Barnavon Y, Wallack MK: Management of the pregnant patient with carcinoma of the breast. Surg Gynecol Obstet 171 (4): 347-52, 1990.
8. Litton JK and Theriault RL. Chapter 65: Breast cancer during pregnancy and subsequent pregnancy in breast cancer survivors, in Harris JR, Lippman ME, Morrow M, Osborne CK. Diseases of the Breast, 5th edition. Lippincott Williams and Wilkins, 2014.
9. Germann N, Goffinet F, Goldwasser F. Anthracyclines during pregnancy: embryo-fetal outcome in 160 patients. Ann Oncol 2004;15:146-150.
10. Johnson PH, Gwyn K, Gordon N, et al. The treatment of pregnant women with breast cancer and the outcomes of the children exposed to chemotherapy in utero [abstract]. J Clin Oncol 2005;23(Suppl 16):Abstract 540.
11. Doll DC, Ringenberg QS, Yarbro JW. Antineoplastic agents and pregnancy. Semin Oncol 1989;16:337-346.
12. Ebert U, Loffler H, Kirch W. Cytotoxic therapy and pregnancy. Pharmacol Ther 1997;74:207-220.
13. Hoover HC Jr: Breast cancer during pregnancy and lactation. Surg Clin North Am 70 (5): 1151-63, 1990.
14. Rugo HS: Management of breast cancer diagnosed during pregnancy. Curr Treat Options Oncol 4 (2): 165-73, 2003.
15. Gwyn K, Theriault R: Breast cancer during pregnancy. Oncology (Huntingt) 15 (1): 39-46; discussion 46, 49-51, 2001.
16. Clark RM, Chua T: Breast cancer and pregnancy: the ultimate challenge. Clin Oncol (R Coll Radiol) 1 (1): 11-8, 1989.
17. Barnavon Y, Wallack MK: Management of the pregnant patient with carcinoma of the breast. Surg Gynecol Obstet 171 (4): 347-52, 1990.
24. Varadarajan R, Edge SB, Yu J, et al. Prognosis of occult breast carcinoma presenting as isolated axillary nodal metastasis. Oncology 2006;71:456-459.
695. Schelfout K, Kersschot E, Van Goethem M, et al. Breast MR imaging in a patient with unilateral axillary lymphadenopathy and unknown primary malignancy. Eur Radiol 2003;13:2128-2132.
25. Joks M, Myśliwiec K,2 and Lewandowski, K. Primary breast lymphoma – a review of the literature and report of three cases. Arch Med Sci. 2011 Feb; 7(1): 27–33.
26. 1. Jeanneret-Sozzi W, Taghian A, Epelbaum R, et al. Primary breast lymphoma: patient profile, outcome and prognostic factors. A multicentre Rare Cancer Network study. BMC Cancer. 2008;8:86.

Paget disease
1. Harris JR, Lippman ME, Morrow M, Osborne CK, editors. Diseases of the Breast. 4th ed. Philadelphia: Lippincott Williams & Wilkins; 2009.
2. Caliskan M, Gatti G, Sosnovskikh I, et al. Paget's disease of the breast: the experience of the European Institute of Oncology and review of the literature. Breast Cancer Research and Treatment 2008;112(3):513–521.
3. Kanitakis J. Mammary and extramammary Paget's disease. Journal of the European Academy of Dermatology and Venereology 2007;21(5):581–590.
4. Kawase K, Dimaio DJ, Tucker SL, et al. Paget's disease of the breast: there is a role for breast-conserving therapy. Annals of Surgical Oncology 2005;12(5):391–397.
5. Marshall JK, Griffith KA, Haffty BG, et al. Conservative management of Paget disease of the breast with radiotherapy: 10- and 15-year results. Cancer 2003;97(9):2142–2149.
6. Sukumvanich P, Bentrem DJ, Cody HS, et al. The role of sentinel lymph node biopsy in Paget's disease of the breast. Annals of Surgical Oncology 2007;14(3):1020–1023.

7. Laronga C, Hasson D, Hoover S, et al. Paget's disease in the era of sentinel lymph node biopsy. American Journal of Surgery 2006;192(4):481–483.
8. Chen CY, Sun LM, Anderson BO. Paget disease of the breast: changing patterns of incidence, clinical presentation, and treatment in the U.S. Cancer 2006;107(7):1448–1458.
9. Ashikari R, Oark K, Huvos AG et al. Paget's disease of the breast. Cancer 1970; 26:680.
10. Nance, FC, DeLoacj DH, Welsh RA et al. Paget's disease of the breast. Ann Surg 1970; 171:864.

Pregnancy

10. Clark RM, Chua T: Breast cancer and pregnancy: the ultimate challenge. Clin Oncol (R Coll Radiol) 1 (1): 11-8, 1989.
11. Harvey JC, Rosen PP, Ashikari R, et al.: The effect of pregnancy on the prognosis of carcinoma of the breast following radical mastectomy. Surg Gynecol Obstet 153 (5): 723-5, 1981.
12. Petrek JA: Pregnancy safety after breast cancer. Cancer 74 (1 Suppl): 528-31, 1994.
13. von Schoultz E, Johansson H, Wilking N, et al.: Influence of prior and subsequent pregnancy on breast cancer prognosis. J Clin Oncol 13 (2): 430-4, 1995.
14. Kroman N, Mouridsen HT: Prognostic influence of pregnancy before, around, and after diagnosis of breast cancer. Breast 12 (6): 516-21, 2003.
15. Malamos NA, Stathopoulos GP, Keramopoulos A, et al.: Pregnancy and offspring after the appearance of breast cancer. Oncology 53 (6): 471-5, 1996 Nov-Dec.
16. Gelber S, Coates AS, Goldhirsch A, et al.: Effect of pregnancy on overall survival after the diagnosis of early-stage breast cancer. J Clin Oncol 19 (6): 1671-5, 2001.
17. Gwyn K, Theriault R: Breast cancer during pregnancy. Oncology (Huntingt) 15 (1): 39-46; discussion 46, 49-51, 2001.
18. Rugo HS: Management of breast cancer diagnosed during pregnancy. Curr Treat Options Oncol 4 (2): 165-73, 2003.

Young

1. https://www.cdc.gov/cancer/breast/young_women/index.htm
2. Tai P, Yu E, Shiels R, et al. Short- and long-term cause-specific survival of patients with inflammatory breast cancer. BMC Cancer 2005; 5:137.
3. Hance KW, Anderson WF, Devesa SS et al. Trends in inflammatory breast carcinoma incidence and survival: the surveillance, epidemiology, and end results program at the National Cancer Institute. J Natl Cancer Inst 2005; 97:966.
4. Anderson WF, Schairer C, Chen BE et al. Epidemiology of inflammatory breast cancer (IBC). Breast Dis 2005-2006; 22:9.
5. https://www.cdc.gov/cancer/breast/young_women/index.htm

6. Valachis A, Tsali L, Pesce LL, Polyzos NP. Safety of pregnancy after primary breast carcinoma in young women: a meta-analysis to overcome bias of healthy mother effect studies. Obstet Gynecol Surv 2010 Dec;65(12):786-93.

14 survivorship

Lymphedema

9. Ozaslan C, Kuru B. Lymphedema after treatment of breast cancer. *Am J Surg* 2004; 187(1): 69-72.

10. Erickson VS, Pearson ML, Ganz PA et al. Arm edema in breast cancer patients. J Natl Cancer Inst 2001;93(2):96.

Follow-up
1. GLOBOCON 2008 Update http:www.iarc.fr/en/media-centre/iarcnews/2011/globocon2008-prev.php
2. DeSantis CE, Lin CC, Mariotto AB et al. Cancer treatment and survivorship statistis, 2014. CA Cancer J Clin 2014; 64(4): 252.
3. Rojas MP, Telaro E, Russo A et al. Follow-up strategies for women treated for early breast cancer. Cochrane Database Syst Rev 2005.
4. Kwan ML, Kushi LH, Weltzien E et al. Alcohol consumption and breast cancer recurrence and survival among women with early0stage breast cancer: the life after cancer epidemiology study. J Clin Oncol 2010; 28(29): 4410.
5. Lyman GH, Greenleee H, Bohike K et al. Integrative therapies during and after breast cancer treatment: ASCO endorsement of the SIO clinical practice guideline. J Clin Oncol 2018; 36(25):2647.

Hot flashes
6. Paddock, Catharine. Acupuncture reduces hot flashes, night sweats in menopause. Medical News oday. MediLexicon, Intl., 25 May 2016.

Fertility; pregnancy after breast cancer
7. Iqbal J, Amir E, Rochon PA et al. Association of the timing of pregnancy with surival in women with breast cancer. JAMA Oncol 2017;3(5):659.
8. Valachis A, Tsali L, Pesce LL et al. Safety of pregnancy after primary breast carcinoma in young
11. Cariati M, Bains SK, Grootendorst MR et al. Adjuvant taxanes and the development of breast cancer-related arm lymphoedema. Br J Surg 2015; 102(9): 1071-1078.
12. McDuff SGR, Mina AI, Brunelle CL et al. Timing of lymphedema after treatment of breast cancer: when are patients most at risk? Int J Radiat Oncol Biol Phys 2019103(1):62.
13. Bloomquist K, Oturai P, Steele ML et al. Heavy-load lifting: Acute response in breast cacer survivors at risk for lymphedema. Med Sci Sports Exer 2018;50(2):187.
14. Moseley Al, Loller NB. Exercise for limb edema: Evidence that it is beneficial. J Lymphoedema 2008;3:51.
15. Schmitz KH, Ahmed Rl, Troxel A, et al. Weight lifting in women with breast-cancer-related lymphedema. N Engl J Med 2009;361(7):664.
16. Ahmed RL, Thomas W, Yee D, Schmitz KH. Randomized controlled trial of weight training and lymphedema in breast cancer survivors. J Clin Oncol 2006;24(18):2765.
17. Ezzo J, Manheimer E, McNeely ML, et al. Manual lymphatic drainage for lymphedema following breast cancer treatment. Cochrane Database Syst Rev 2015.
18. Didem K, Ufuk YS, and Sumre A. The comparison of two different physiotherapy methods in treatment of lymphedema after breast surgery. Breast Cancer Res Treat 2005;93(1):49.
19. Dayes IS, Whelan TJ, Julian JA et al. Randomized tiral of decongestive lymphatic drainage for the treatment of lymphedema in women with breast cancer. J Clin Oncol 2013;31(30):3758-63.
20. Ezzo J, Manheimer E, McNeely ML, et al. Manual lymphatic drainage for lymphedema following breast cancer treatment. Cochrane Database Syst Rev 2015.
21. DiSipio T, Rye S, Newman B, Hayes S. Incidence of unilateral arm lymphoedema after breast cancer: a systematic review and meta-analysis. Lancet Oncol 2013;14(6):500.
22. Cancer. 2012 Mar 15;118(6):1710-7. doi: 10.1002/cncr.26459. Epub 2011 Sep 1. Pretreatment fertility counseling and fertility preservation improve quality of life in reproductive age women with cancer.
23. Letourneau J, Ebbel E, Katz P. Pretreatment fertility counseling and fertility preservation improve quality of life in reproductive age women with cancer. Cancer. 2012;118(6):1710-7.

Made in the USA
Las Vegas, NV
07 April 2021